Solution Recovery from Eating Distress

Frederike Jacob

BT Press

First published June 2001
Published by BT Press
17 Avenue Mansions, Finchley Road, London NW3 7AX

© Frederike Jacob 2001

Design by Alex Gollner

No part of this publication may be reproduced, stored in a retrieval system, or transmitted in any form or by any means, electronic, mechanical, photocopying, recording or otherwise, without the permission of the copyright owner.

ISBN 1 871697 76 X

Contents

Foreword	5
Letter to the Reader	6
Introduction	8
1. What is Solution-Focused Therapy?	9
2. What Are Eating Disorders?	33
3. The Treatment	48
4. Case Studies	77
5. Any Questions?	140
Bibliography	149
Useful Addresses	151

To my clients

Foreword

Frederike Jacob has written a milestone book both for solution focused brief therapy and the field of eating disorders. Solution-focused brief therapy is a generic "all purpose" approach and eating disorders are seen as a very specialist subject. As the title of the book asks: Can the two be reconciled? Frederike Jacob clearly thinks so and argues her case well. She provides a succinct description of solution focused therapy alongside an equally succinct description of the variety of forms an eating disorder might take. The matter-of-factness of these descriptions reduces the mystique of both: solution-focused brief therapy is seen as a perfectly logical and straightforward process and eating disorders are seen as ways of behaving that can be changed.

On the other hand, the potentially fatal consequences of an eating disorder are not ignored and throughout the book close attention is paid to clients' safety and to ways the professional might promote and safeguard this. It is this responsible attitude towards the client's health and safety that creates the real possibility of developing a non-medicalised form of treatment. For many struggling with eating problems this development will open new possibilities for a better life.

Frederike Jacob's practical approach to her subject is no better demonstrated than in the descriptions of her work with clients. In these the problem, the process, the thinking and the outcome are all clearly spelled out, some in the form of word by word transcripts. Case by case, a way to do solution-focused brief therapy unfolds.

When Steve de Shazer, the person most responsible for articulating solution-focused ideas, wrote his first books he was criticised for his "cookbook" style: "You can't learn therapy from books!" was the cry. Yet tens if not hundreds of thousands of therapists all over the world have found a way to make de Shazer's ideas their own. This is a book that follows the de Shazer tradition – it is a book from which the reader can learn. That means it is worth reading.

Chris Iveson
Brief Therapy Practice
London

LETTER TO THE READER

Ipswich, 10th December 2000.

Dear Reader,

As I start to write this book, I project my thoughts towards when it is finished and has found its way into your hands and I wonder ...
Why did you choose to pick up this particular book?
Were you intrigued by its title, or by the cover?
Are you a professional, trying to support someone in recovery from eating distress? If so, do you find people with eating disorders "impossible to work with"? Maybe you have a friend or relative who suffers, or you may even have (had) difficulties with food yourself.
Or are you simply wondering what solution-focused therapy is all about?
I guess any or all of the above could apply to you and I am aware that I could not possibly do justice to everyone who has a link with eating disorders. Although this book deals with therapeutic interventions in particular, I hope that whatever your background, you will be inspired and encouraged by what you read.
I am a solution-focused therapist with a specific interest in helping clients overcome their difficulties with food. I have worked in this field as an independent practitioner since 1997, and after I presented a workshop in Finland at the European Brief Therapy Conference in 2000, I was invited to write this book.
My way of working has been shaped by carefully monitoring my clients' progress and by doing more of what they tell me is useful and supportive. I did not set out to produce a comprehensive textbook on the intricacies of eating disorders, only to write from my experience as a therapist. The examples I present come from my own practice. They may or may not fit your particular circumstances or therapeutic model, but maybe you will consider and experiment with some of the ideas by moulding them to fit your individual way of working.
I would like to point out that although the techniques and interventions described here are used to combat eating distress, they are in no way restricted to dealing with that problem alone. I find they lend themselves equally well to helping clients overcome a spectrum of problems such as depression, relationship difficulties, anxiety, substance or alcohol misuse and school- or work-related stress.

My aim is to convey a message of hope. Too often books, TV or radio programmes and journalistic articles cover the "down-side" of eating distress. This has resulted in a negative attitude to the problem and towards those who try to recover.

When I am asked what I do for a living, my reply is often met with a sympathetic look or a shake of the head. People say: "Eating disorders.... Gosh, that must be difficult!" or, "Those clients are so resistant, so manipulative, aren't they?" or, "They never recover ... what a depressing job you have. You must suffer from burn-out!" My experience is quite the opposite, and this may have something to do with the therapeutic model I work with. Initially, I underwent psychodynamic counselling training, and in such traditional therapy the problem is the central issue. Causes, consequences and maintaining factors are explored in detail. This makes for lengthy – and in my view depressing – therapy, in which many clients report "becoming stuck".

When I was introduced to solution-focused therapy I learned that, in contrast, the therapist is interested in those times the problem is (slightly) less oppressive, and will specifically explore occasions when clients feel they can cope a little better. The therapist is also curious to know how clients envisage a future when the problem has disappeared, or when they are better able to manage it. My colleagues and I have discovered that this motivational way of working moves clients on and creates a sense of optimism. In my experience this not only prevents clients getting stuck, but also safeguards therapists against burning out. These issues will be addressed in more detail later.

I hope this book will help to explode the myth that people with eating disorders are "difficult clients" and I welcome this opportunity to show the courage, integrity, creativity and humour that I have seen as predominant character traits among my clients. To protect their anonymity, I have changed their names and identifiable details.

I am indebted to all my clients for what they have taught me over the years, and am grateful to those who allowed me to share their stories with you.

With best wishes,

F.J.

INTRODUCTION

The 1980s and '90s saw a marked increase in eating disorders, and this trend is set to continue into the new century. We can assume that more people will seek help to overcome such problems. Based on solution-focused principles, this book offers practitioners ideas to promote recovery.

Chapter One briefly explains the solution-focused approach. I have illustrated the techniques and interventions with snippets from sessions with clients, because they are particularly relevant to working with eating disorders. If this is your first encounter with this therapeutic model you may wish to obtain more in-depth explanations of solution-focused therapy (SFT) and how it can be used in other fields. To this end there are some recommendations for further reading at the end of the book.

Chapter Two concerns what is generally understood by the term "eating disorders". Although in most cases expertise is not required, my clients often say that it is helpful when therapists have some understanding of what is happening to them. Alongside this, I think that a broad knowledge of the associated signs, symptoms and, in more serious cases the dangerous side-effects, will make for safer practice.

Chapter Three talks about the treatment currently on offer, and places solution-focused therapy within other therapeutic paradigms. It shows how solution-focused interventions can be used to combat eating disorders, and there are several examples that show how it works in practice.

I have a keen interest in finding out what it is that works for clients. At the end of each session we discuss what has been particularly useful, and evaluate our work in the final session. Over the years, this feedback has shaped and developed specific concepts, ideas and ways of working, and some of these are included in this section.

Chapter Four examines a number of case studies to give a more in-depth insight into how solution-focused interventions are used in practice and the final chapter is devoted to answering questions I am most commonly asked.

I.

WHAT IS SOLUTION-FOCUSED THERAPY?

How it started
The solution-focused approach was conceptualised by Insoo Kim Berg and Steve de Shazer in Milwaukee, USA, in the early 1980s. While traditional therapy involved deep explorations into the client's problem-saturated past, practitioners discovered that their clients made significant progress by talking about a "preferred future". Inviting clients to describe how they pictured life once they had overcome their problem resulted in a consistently favourable outcome. The work involved looking for exceptions (occasions when the problem was easier to handle), being future-oriented, and collaboratively devising small, achievable goals. New coping strategies and solutions replaced the problem thinking in which so many clients had become stuck.

With their team at the Brief Family Therapy Center (de Shazer 1998) they subjected their initial findings to rigorous tests. They honed, refined and perfected specific interventions until they came up with a way of working which they named Solution-Focused Brief Therapy (SFBT).

Their practical concepts are now widely used in the therapeutic field, but are found to be equally effective in other settings, e.g. management consultation, career counselling, in schools and nursing, to name but a few.

A bit of theory
Solution-focused therapy belongs to the "constructionist" school,[†] where therapy becomes a dialogue in which both partners construct the problem and the solution. It is a "language game" (Friedman, 1993), in which clients tell and re-tell their stories using language which reshapes the social reality in which they live. In effect, language creates reality.

---

† Constructionism states that meaning is known only through social interaction and negotiation. We have no direct access to objective truth, independent of our linguistically constructed versions of reality. (O'Connell, 1998)

According to Wittgenstein (Grayling, 1996), whose philosophical thinking supports solution-focused therapy, the language we are "in" provides both *possibilities* and *limitations* for what we can understand and how we understand it. The possibilities lie in the richness of language and its capacity closely to convey personal meanings to others. But alongside this co-exist limitations: we all live according to individual internal belief-systems and experiences. Therefore it is impossible really to understand what goes on within another person's mind. As de Shazer says, the optimum we can work towards is: *"How can I best mis-understand you?"* (Friedman, 1993).

For example, people with eating disorders often hear comments such as, "Why don't you just eat something" (anorexia nervosa) or, "Just leave those chocolates alone and have an apple instead!" (compulsive binge eating or bulimia nervosa). These are classic examples of "missing the point". Were it that simple, there would be no problem, and my colleagues and I would be out of a job!

The *"How can I best mis-understand you"* concept involves saying something like, "I can't possibly understand what it's like to be in your tight spot, and how could I, since I am me and you are you. But you can help me to get as close as I can, so we can join forces and try to get out of it together." This opens the way to the collaborative work that is described in this book

Problem v solution

As its name implies, solution-focused therapy concentrates on solutions and preferred futures in preference to problems. We amplify clients' strengths and abilities we believe co-exist alongside their dilemmas and difficulties. We look for evidence in the client's story that proves that however bad the circumstances, he or she is already doing something which prevents the problem worsening. In an empowering exercise, the client is encouraged to do more of what works.

Therapy is still regarded by many as being about an in-depth exploration of difficulties. Traditionalists think that getting to know what's wrong, coming to grips with it and facing up to it are essential stages that need to be completed before clients can move forward. This is thought that to be a "cathartic" process. However, those committed to solution-focused therapy think that problem-focused work may lead to feelings of inadequacy and hopelessness. If you are new to solution-focused therapy, it may be surprising to know that successful work has been done without referring to the problem at all!

The difference between problem- and solution-focused work can be illustrated by imagining the therapy room to be a theatre set, where the leading actors are Problem and Solution. They are supported by Client and Therapist.

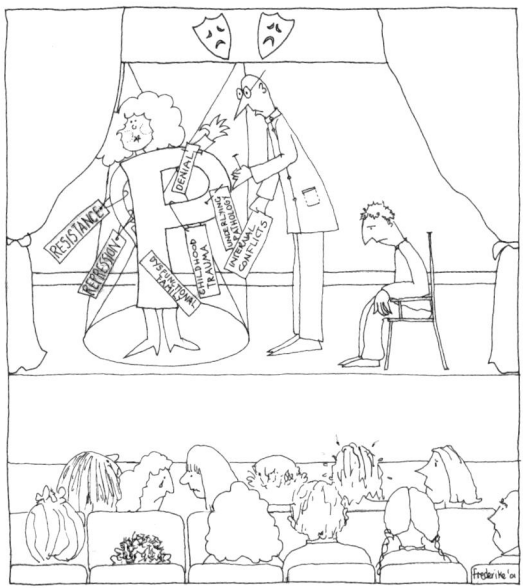

Client and Therapist stare into the middle of the room where, bathed in floodlights, Problem holds centre stage. Problem is examined closely from every angle, turned this way and that to get a better look. Its origins are excavated and much of the discussion evolves around psychodynamic interactions related to events that took place in childhood and the people who are causing or have caused the client distress. The therapist hypothesises and the client is awe-struck in the presence of this Very Learned Person.

Meanwhile, Problem is basking in all the attention. It puffs up self-importantly, and becomes more real by the minute. Like a magnet it attracts labels, such as Depression, Underlying Pathologies, Systemic Dysfunction, Resistance, Collusion, Psychodynamic Discords, Repression, Denial, Regression, Manipulative Attitudes and so on.

Finally, with hushed voice and grave face, Therapist proclaims his diagnosis.

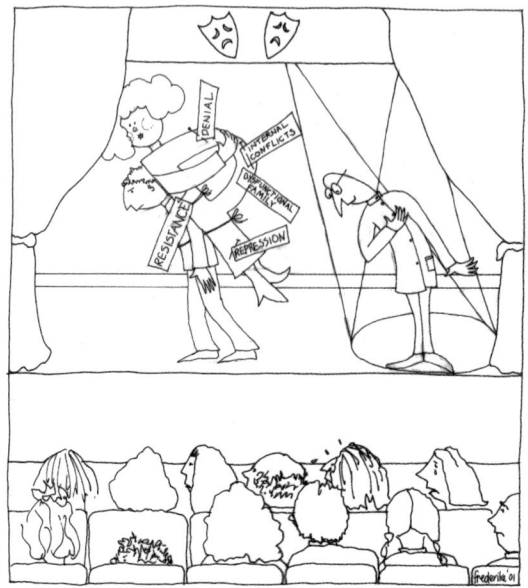

Client exits. Bent under the weight of Problem, he is even more convinced than before that he is in very grave trouble. The stage is set for long-term therapy.

Curtain down, interval, then back to your seats for Act Two.

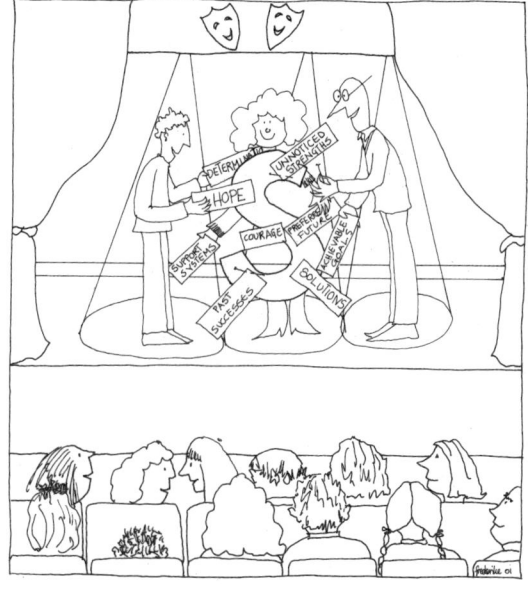

Client and Therapist are in conversation while Solution stands in the centre of the stage. The discussion is very different to that of Act One. There is little talk about Problem. What is focused upon instead are the times when Client was a little better able to cope, and who was there to give support. The discussion projects Client's thoughts towards a preferred future, which evolves around what life will be like when Problem has disappeared. Together, Therapist and Client find evidence of exceptions, the times that Problem appears to be less powerful, and Client is already doing something positive.

Solution has magnetic powers too: it attracts evidence of character traits such as hopefulness, confidence, capability, creativity, resilience, staying-power, self-esteem, optimism, assertiveness, self-control. ... These enable Client to see that he has some ability to do something to make his problem a little less arduous.

Therapist and Client collaboratively puff up Solution and at the end of the session Client leaves the stage upright, with a bounce in his step, supported and empowered by Solution and also more optimistic, knowing that Problem can be defeated in the shortest possible time.

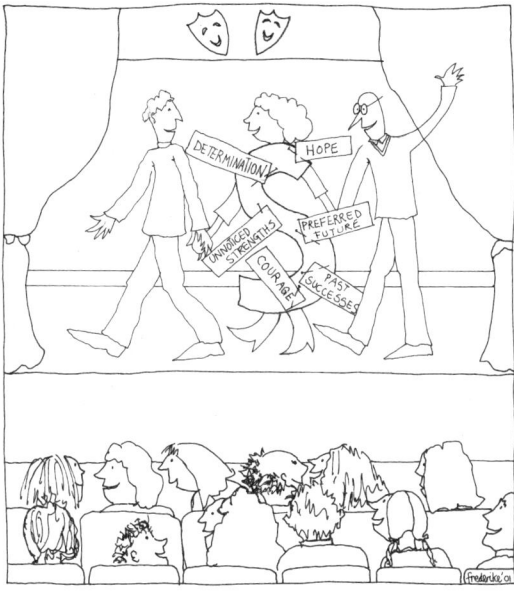

How it works

Solution-focused therapists do not believe that current difficulties can be resolved by identifying "underlying issues", nor by lengthy and in-depth explorations of the problem, its causes, and how it is maintained within interactional patterns. They assume instead that clients become empowered and achieve change more quickly by constructing and developing solutions.

Another assumption is that in our world nothing is ever constant, so there will be times that the problem is not as bad as usual. These times are called "exceptions", and they are focused upon and amplified in the therapeutic process. Take one of my clients, for example, who exclaimed that she was "constantly vomiting". That statement immediately tickled my curiosity. I wondered aloud, "What ... *always*?" Even when you are asleep? Even when you hang out the washing? Even when you walk your children to school? Even while you're in the shower?"

What transpired was that she vomited on average twice or three times a day. It may be tempting to follow up this information with questions such as, "What leads up to those times that you vomit?" or, "What is your relationship like with the people who frustrate you so much that you want to vomit?" But solution-focused therapy would focus on the times that the client did *not* vomit, to highlight a wealth of coping strategies and support structures that are already in place.

Considering language to be the medium for change, meaning is co-constructed in conversation. The therapist will empathise, and closely follow the client's agenda, while the non-pathologising approach helps to create options and possibilities. In a nutshell, there is no need to make interpretations or speculations regarding the role and function of eating, restricting or purging behaviours. Instead, the usefulness of the eating disorder is challenged and solutions are built to move towards the client's preferred future (McFarland 1995).

Many clients initially present with multiple, inter-related problems and it is essential to establish early on what will be the main goal of therapy. Staying focused can be a very tricky business. Yet it is imperative not to get waylaid by unrelated, juicy stories, because in the end these only serve to muddy the therapeutic waters and make for a confusing process. In other words, if the client's goal is to have a more regular eating pattern, it is not much use getting sidetracked into trying to improve her relationship with crotchety great-aunt Agatha. Furthermore, clients report that when positive change is made in one area, other aspects of their lives benefit as well. I have found that as a client grows more assertive in relationship to the eating disorder, the attitude towards great-aunt Agatha will improve too. It is a great economy: two positive changes for the price of one!

Solution-focused therapy can be considered a directional way of working. By asking specific solution- and future-oriented questions, the therapist ensures that problems are not dwelt upon. At the same time, it is commonly accepted that it can be therapeutic for the client to share how bad things have been. Any therapist worth her salt will give the client space to talk about difficulties. But in contrast to analytical therapy, which looks for deficits and hidden pathology, the solution-focused therapist acknowledges the problem and sympathises with how difficult things must have been, whilst amplifying the resources, coping-strategies and strengths which have enabled the client to survive.

John (39), a businessman, had been through a particularly nasty divorce, closely followed by redundancy. This crushed his self-esteem to such an extent that he resorted to comfort eating. He put on a massive amount of weight and at about 140 kilos he was self-conscious and deeply unhappy. He spent the first few sessions pouring his heart out, telling me how bad things had been. I empathised, marvelled at his staying power, and picked up on useful coping strategies he had employed to survive.

By the fourth session he recognised that he had dwelt upon his problems long enough and it was time to start looking forward. When therapy was finished he said that being able to let off steam in those first sessions had been particularly helpful. It had made him realise that he did have a "survival streak" in him which made him feel less victimised by his ex-wife, ex-boss and the eating disorder.

Solution-Focused *Brief* Therapy?
The team in Milwaukee who first thought up the concept, named the model Solution-Focused *Brief* Therapy, and many therapists follow this example. With the greatest respect to them, I like to refer to my work as "solution-focused therapy" because, having worked for two years with some clients, I feel the term solution-focused *brief* therapy would be wrong for the specific work that I do.

Many solution-focused colleagues claim successful outcomes after an average of two-point-something sessions, no matter what the problem was. Although few of my clients finish therapy that quickly, the majority make significant improvements in under ten meetings.

The number of sessions that clients require varies and largely depends on the severity of the difficulty needing to be overcome, the motivation of the client, and the progress they have made before therapy begins. Each session is set up as an individual unit and at the end we assess how useful our work has been. In contrast to other therapeutic models, there is no pre-set contract and the client decides on the number and frequency of visits. My clients often have a few weekly sessions, but as soon as possible these are spread further apart. This acknowledges that most clients can function at a good enough level between sessions and that they can make changes without intensive and long-term therapeutic support.

When clients present with chronic forms of the illness for which longer-term therapy may be indicated, I use the principle that if they find it beneficial and there are signs of progress, we continue our working alliance, bearing in mind that we use only the absolute minimum amount of sessions necessary.

In our present economic climate where cost-effectiveness is high on the agenda, the prospect of long-term therapy is an unattractive one. Miller, Hubble and Duncan (1997) quote research which shows that solution-focused therapy tends to be briefer than other therapies. This considerably reduces the financial strain often caused by traditional, weekly, open-ended work. Although on the face of it this may not seem so good for the therapist's bank balance, clients appreciate this approach and will recommend the service to others. This makes for a steady flow of clients, and in turn, yields a reasonable income.

The term "brief" is often mistakenly interpreted as "quick fix" or "plaster on the wound" therapy. Trying to complete therapy in the fewest possible sessions without regard for the client's needs, or being "solution-forced" (O'Connell, 1998), could indeed result in an unsatisfactory outcome. However, research shows that solution-focused therapy has similar outcomes to other models and my statistics also show that many clients continue to make progress after therapy has finished.

Past v future

Solution-focused therapy is future oriented, and it is often said that we do not need to know where we have come from in order to know where we want to get to (de Shazer). In other words, it is not necessary to rake over our problem-laden past in order to create a better future. By asking directive questions, the therapist leads a client's train of thought to the life ahead when he or she is better able to cope. In the first session, clients describe in minute detail the differences in their life when the problem which has brought them to therapy has miraculously been resolved. This breaks away from the past and the problem, and gives both client and therapist a clear idea of what the client wishes to achieve. Between them, they work out small achievable steps to bring about change.

As early as the first session, the therapist addresses ending the working relationship by asking, "How will we know when therapy has finished? What will you be doing that will indicate to us that our work is done?" This creates the hope and expectation that some change will take place and helps create a goal towards which they can work.

Liz, an ex-client and research participant, described the change of focus from past problem to future solution as follows:

> I remember our first session. ... I was astounded to start with. I had never been in therapy and I imagined to be really nurtured and you going, 'There, there,' and we'd talk about how awful it all was. And I do remember you sitting down, putting your notepad on your lap, and we just launched straight into it! [laughs] This just threw me totally because that was not what I was expecting at all! But I came away feeling like I had travelled more in one hour than I had in ages. Because I wasn't allowed to sit and dwell on it all, which in hindsight was good, because I knew about that side of it anyway, and there was no point in going over it again.
>
> There was a sense of momentum ... so much progress had been made

in one session. You'd hit the nail on the head! The fact that I wanted to move on. This approach was so much more against the problem: leaving it behind. And, "This is how we are going forward." So it missed the whole chunk in the middle, where I had got stuck.

Power, equality and responsibility.
Clients generally start therapy because they want something to change. They can expect an approach which respects that they know their own limitations, hopes and desires. We say the client is considered to be "expert in their life", while the therapist is expert in his or her profession. In SFT these fields of expertise are dovetailed together to form a working relationship based on equality and mutual respect.

Equality is fostered by giving the client's expertise as much weight as the therapist's. I think this is in contrast to the hierarchical approach of psychodynamics. Freud wrote that analysis is "a situation in which there is a superior and a subordinate" (Masson, 1993). That is, the therapist is superior, the client inferior. It seems to me that he was unable to transcend the dominant discourses of his day, which blinded him to what the client was telling him, or what the client wanted to achieve. Solution-focused practitioners choose to demystify the therapeutic process by explaining to clients exactly what the counselling entails, so that they can give their informed consent (O'Connell, 1998). An SFT therapist uses language that is easily understood (no professional jargon) and will adjust the choice of words to a client's vocabulary.

Whatever field we work in, it is generally recognised that the final responsibility for change has to be with the clients, who are considered persons of free will. Therefore, in terms of eating disorders, irrespective of the thoughts or expertise of the therapist, *clients* will ultimately decide whether and what they will eat.

Those of us in a professional capacity who support people in eating distress need to familiarise ourselves with the professional and ethical guidelines of the appropriate professional body. For instance, the British Association for Counselling and Psychotherapy (BACP) states that if a therapist is concerned about the safety of a client, e.g. the client is in danger of self-harming (which includes issues of underfeeding), the rule of confidentiality must be broken. When I am worried about a client's physical or emotional state I may suggest he or she approaches a doctor for additional support. On rare occasions, I have overruled the client's wish not to get the doctor involved, and voiced my concern to their GP. It would have been unsafe practice and unethical not to have done so, and this was clearly explained to the client. This may or may not have an effect on the therapeutic relationship; clients may terminate therapy as a result. Therapists are free to do so too, if they feel they cannot provide adequate support, and it may be helpful if the therapist can suggest alternative forms of help.

On occasions I am invited to work as part of a multi-disciplinary team. When I find myself in such a situation I make it clear to all involved that I work in a transparent way: I try to co-write any reports with my clients, or at least get their approval on what I have written before it is sent. I also inform my client of any communication I receive about them and if at all possible, invite them to attend meetings where their treatment is discussed. This way of working promotes trust and increases the client's involvement and responsibility for their recovery.

In extreme cases, e.g. when clients become a danger to themselves or society, or when they have become emaciated to the extent that intravenous nutrition becomes essential, medical professionals may decide to section the client, that is, admit them to a (psychiatric) hospital against their wishes at which point therapy may have to be suspended.

Solution-Focused Tools and Interventions

Several aspects need to be present for therapy to be regarded as solution focused. They are described here in the order they are generally used within a first session.

Pre-session change

SFT acknowledges that change is ongoing whether clients are receiving therapy or not. Giving attention to pre-session change empowers the client because it proves that they can instigate change independently, even before therapy has started. Pre-session change is not uncommon. Clients often report that, "Once I made the decision to do something about it I started to feel a little better." The therapist can follow this up with affirmations and curiosity about what, as a result of "feeling a little better", has changed in the client's life. I have found that outcome tends to improve if clients are able to identify pre-session change.

We can take this a step further by telling clients that we are *expecting* some pre-session change. When they make their first appointment – either in person or by telephone – they are invited to start looking for small positive changes and/or times that the problem is less oppressive.

> "Between now and when we meet, I would like you to spot any small changes or times that you feel you are a little more able to cope. This will give us something to go on in our first session."

If appointments are arranged by someone other than the therapist, e.g. a colleague or receptionist, they could say this to every new client:

> "Between now and the day of your appointment, the therapist would like you to …" etc. (Berg, 1993)

The following examples illustrate the significance of focusing on pre-session change. As soon as the initial details are taken, Lily (24) launches straight into problem description. She has had bulimia for seven years. It has made her very grumpy and has prevented her from going out and socialising. The therapist explains that she would like to ask a few questions first before they talk about the problem.

T: Do you remember our telephone conversation last week?
L: Hmm, yeah …
T: I invited you to look out for any positive changes. Have you noticed anything different that you were pleased about?
L: I felt really good after I spoke to you on the telephone, you know … that I'd really started something. But later I had a big row with my boyfriend. Normally I would have gone to the kitchen and stuffed my face, but this time I had a cup of tea instead.
T: That's great! How did you do that?
L: Well, I just thought, "No. I've made a start now, I'm sticking to it!"
T: How did that make you feel?
L: Well … good actually, 'cos I didn't have to beat myself up over scoffing.
T: Great! And as a result, what were you able to do differently?

The therapist takes the emphasis away from the problem, and focuses on what has been going well. This turns the conversation in a positive, empowering direction.

The next example describes the start of a session with a woman (20), who had suffered from anorexia nervosa since she was sixteen.

T: Did you notice anything different, anything positive since you made your appointment?
C: [Sighs] Not much, really. No … nothing.
T: So the eating … it's difficult. Have there been times you were able to eat anything at all?
C: Yeah … I did, at my Gran's birthday party. There was a barbecue and I ate some salad.
T: Wow … you just did that?
C: Yeah, nothing much really.…
T: But you *did* it!
C: Yeah, and in front of my family as well! [Looks triumphant]
T: Gosh, brilliant. What happened there? How did you do it?
C: I dunno, really, saw them all tucking in … hmm. Yeah, that surprised them.
T: I bet!

In this case, the therapist amplifies what the client considers insignificant, and the client begins to feel good about her small step. This encourages her to "do more of what works."

We have to be aware that some clients have not experienced positive pre-session change, and to adapt our questions accordingly. We understand that however bad things are for the client, they could always be a fraction worse, and we are curious to find out what the client is already doing to prevent things from deteriorating, e.g.

T: Have you noticed any positive changes since we made this appointment?
C: No. Nothing.
T: Nothing at all?
C: No. If anything, things have got worse....
T: I see.
C: Hmm. I can't control it *at all!*
T: Can you explain a little more?
C: Yeah. I've now started vomiting after most meals.
T: After most meals. I see ... how come it's not after *every* meal?

This leads the conversation into focusing on exceptions. The client had come in feeling totally hopeless and now faces the reality that at times he does have *some* control over the binge-vomit habit.

Problem-free talk
Many clients have the pre-conceived idea that they have come to therapy to unearth "deep and meaningful" reasons for their problem. If they are fixed on this course, they may need some encouragement to set their burden aside for a while. The therapist explains that she first wants to get to know the *client* rather than the *problem* and invites them to share what is typical about them (e.g. hobbies, family, friends, interests, job) *without* referring to the reasons for seeking therapy. When clients have been entrenched in the problem this is sometimes hard to do, but it is a vital aspect of therapy as it begins to take the focus away from the problem. It may be necessary to say something like this:

"Is it OK with you if we put the problem that brought you here to one side for the moment? I'd like to get to know you a little.... What is typical about you? Your family, or friends? What are the things you like doing, hobbies ... that sort of thing? We'll talk about those, and we can get back to the problem a little later."

Problem definition
Sometimes clients can get so enthusiastic about the things they like doing that they forget about the problem that brought them in the first place. In this case the "prob-

lem definition" part can be skipped.

However, for some it is therapeutic to talk about what has happened to them and they may need to describe a problem in detail. This is of course respected, but rather than analysing the cause, the therapist listens intently to the story and looks for resources that have helped the client to cope and survive. Questions are asked in a way that teaches both client and therapist about the actual function of the problem within the client's reality.

T: So you binge-vomit, say, three or four times a day?
C: Yeah.
T: And you say this is useful.
C: Yeah. Eating is good, feeling full is bad. Feeling empty is good.

Or:
C: Thinking about food all the time makes me feel safe, because then I don't have to think about when I was bullied.

Or:
C: I need to feel clean.... Ever since he raped me, I just need to feel clean. I scrub and scrub myself so I am clean on the outside, and then I take 20 laxatives because they help me feel clean on the inside.

The therapist now has an idea of the function of the problem. With the utmost respect for where the client is coming from, solution-focused questions will be asked in order to discover and devise alternative, less destructive ways to feel "good" or "safe" or "clean".

The Miracle Question
Many solution-focused therapists go on to ask the "Miracle Question". This helps clients focus on what life will be like when the problem is more manageable or has been resolved.

The therapist asks the following question: "Imagine that when you go to sleep, a miracle happens and your problem has disappeared. When you wake up the next morning, you don't know the miracle has happened, as you were fast asleep.... What will be the first sign that tells you the miracle has happened?"

Most of my clients say, "I won't immediately think about food."

This answer needs further exploration and the next question could be this: "So what will you be thinking about instead?" If they say, "I will be happy," I would want to know, "What is that like? How do you 'do' happy? Imagine you were watching yourself on video, what would you see yourself doing that tells you that you are happy? What will you notice yourself doing differently?" (O'Hanlon, 1997) The questions, "Who will be the first to notice?" "What will their reaction be?" "How will you respond to that?" and "What will others notice?" bring the client's environment and support structure into focus.

Rich descriptions are gathered about how the "Miracle Day" develops from first waking up to going to bed at night. This enables the client to paint a detailed picture of what life could be like without the problem. I like to spend as long as possible on this question, milking it for all it is worth. As some clients have been struggling with an eating disorder for years it can take a little time for them to get the hang of the solution-focused way of working. Some gentle coaching may be required.

What follows is a fairly typical scenario. Caroline (18) has suffered from bulimia nervosa for four years. She has come to see me because she says she is "sick and tired of the whole thing" (we laughed about the pun). Now she "just wants to get better." The Miracle Question is asked:

T: What will be the first thing you notice that's different as you open your eyes?
C: Hmm. I don't know ... [T waits patiently]
C: You ask weird questions!
T: I do, you're right ... [Continues to wait].
C: Hmm. I suppose I'd not wake up thinking about food.
T: Hmm?
C: Can't think of anything else.
T: OK. So ... if you're not thinking about food, what else will you be thinking about?
C: Now, that I really *don't* know!
T: Another tricky question! [Laughter]
C: Hmm. What would I be thinking about instead? I suppose about what I'd be doing that day?
T: Is it a working day or a weekend day?
C: Definitely a weekend.
T: So there you are, in your bed, it's the week-end ... just opened your eyes thinking, "What shall I do today?"
C. Hmm.
T: How do you feel?
C: I wouldn't feel so down and depressed.
T: Oh, OK. So how *do* you feel?
C: Mm. Dunno, really. Hmm ... I'd feel happy ... and relaxed.
T: Imagine you could watch this scene on video ... can you describe to me what you see yourself doing differently? How do you *see* that you are happy and relaxed?

C: I'd be snuggled up, with a smile on my face. Yeah. And … and I'd probably think, "I'll ring one of my friends and go to the beach."
T: Mm, good idea! Is it a sunny day?
C: Too right it is! Yeah, lovely. A day by the beach.
T: So then what happens. Do you jump out of bed? Do you snuggle down a little longer?
C: No, I'll jump out. [Shows jumping action with hands]
T: Full of bounce!
C: Yeah, full of energy.
T: And then what will you do differently on this Miracle Day?
C: I'll have a shower
T: And what's different about that?
C: I won't be pinching and punching my stomach…
T: What do you do instead?
C: I can stand under the shower for ages and …
T: And…. What else?
C: And I really like my body. I can bear to look in the mirror. I will have lost some weight.
T: Mm! And then?
C: Yeah. Then I'll get dressed and have some breakfast.
T: Do you choose anything different to wear?
C: Yes. I won't wear drab or black.
T: OK, so instead what will you choose?
C: Some bright colours, my shocking pink T-shirt.
T: Aha! To match your hair! [Client has bright pink streak in her hair]
C: [Laughs] Yeah! Cool!
T: OK. And then, you say, you have breakfast. What will you have on this Miracle Day?
C: I won't have rubbish.
T: So what will you go for?
C: Hmm … some cereal,
T: Anything else? Miracle Day, remember? A special treat, perhaps?
C: Oh, yes! I'll treat myself to some of that nice expensive orange juice with bits in.
T: You make my mouth water!
C: And mine! [Laughter]
Therapist and client continue to explore the Miracle Day in detail.

This example illustrates that clients may find it difficult to change their problem-focused train of thought into solution-focused thinking. The Miracle Question is often responded to by, "I don't know". Don't be disheartened by this. It does not necessarily mean that you have asked the wrong question, rather that it is an unexpected one and the client needs a little time to formulate an answer. Patiently waiting for that answer often does the trick, but if the client makes it clear that the Miracle Question is totally off limits, you can try rephrasing it or letting the client change the course of the conversation. It may be that more time is needed to tell you how awful things are, or have been.

Another common finding is that many clients know exactly what will *no longer* be happening (see above: I won't be thinking about food, I won't feel down and depressed, I won't wear drab clothes), but cannot answer the question, "What will happen *instead?*" The therapist will try to elicit *positive* alternatives, as the example above showed. "So you won't wear drab clothes ... what will you choose instead?" is followed by what Caroline would prefer to wear. Systematically, negative thought patterns are turned into positive ones. Often it is useful to rephrase tentative possibilities prefaced by "would", "should" or "could" into more definite ones, such as "will", "shall" and "can". For instance, the client's "I *would* choose to wear bright colours" is repeated as, "So you *will* wear bright colours," while "I *could* try to eat breakfast" becomes, "You *can* try to have some breakfast."

The example shows how quickly a change of attitude can happen. Caroline uses "would" in the first few sentences, but soon begins to respond to the therapist's reframing. She is beginning to map out a future for herself which becomes more achievable as the session progresses.

I have found that it is important to let the client do the work. I may have fantastic and exciting ideas of what might be happening on the Miracle Day (I admit I can get quite carried away), but if they do not fit the client's, she will feel ill-understood and an opportunity to gain trust may be squandered.

Caroline's story also begins to introduce the all-important aspect of self-nurturing. Clients with eating disorders often have a low opinion of themselves and feel they do not deserve a treat. But a few minutes into the work, Caroline is already able, in theory, to allow herself some nice expensive "orange juice with bits in." These kinds of conversation begin to turn ideas into achievable realities that can be experimented with in between sessions.

With some clients it would simply be inappropriate to talk about a miracle, so a few variations that give similar responses are these:

"Imagine we have a crystal ball and we can see a year ahead. Things have changed in the best way possible. What can you see? What is different? Who was the first to notice? What was their reaction? What happened as a consequence? "

or:

"Say in a few months from now we bump into each other in town, and you tell me that you have overcome the problem. What will you say has changed? Who noticed the difference?"

Scales

Next, scales (not the weighing kind!) are used to assess progress. The therapist draws a horizontal line. A zero is put on the far left end and represents the worst things could get, or indeed could ever be. The number 10 is put on the right and represents the Miracle Day. Clients are then asked to identify where they are on this scale. Many solution-focused therapists, including myself, have noticed that clients place themselves higher if the scaling exercise is done after rather than before the Miracle Question, and sometimes clients can identify a shift within the session.

"When I came in I was at 2, but now I feel at 5!"

This can be followed up with, "How did you do that?" "What will you be able to do as a result?" "How long do you think you'd be able to stay at 5?" "Who else will notice that you are now at 5?" "What will their reaction be?" "And what is your response?" etc.

Some clients describe themselves as being below zero, e.g. "I'm minus 20". It pays to take this seriously, and at the same time being curious: "How come you're not at minus 21?"

If clients indicate a number above zero, questions such as, "How did you manage to get to that level?" or "How come you are not any lower?" emphasise that they are already preventing things from getting worse. They can then be encouraged to do more of what works to help things get a little better. The scale is used in every session to measure how far along the client is in recovery, and to explore what more needs to be done to move up the scale.

> Claire (13) has recently found it difficult to eat, particularly in company. She has lost some weight and is beginning to withdraw from the activities she used to enjoy.

T: So where would you put yourself on the scale today?
C: At a 2.
T: Have you ever felt lower than a 2?
C: Yeah, I've been as low as 0.
T: That sounds pretty bad.... How did you get yourself to a 2?
C: My fiends helped, talking to them ... my teachers helped ... they kept an eye on me.
T: So you enlisted the help of your teachers and your friends to get up to 2. That sounds clever! I wonder, what would life look like at a 3?

C: [Thinks for a while] I'd be eating a little more.
T: Eating a little more would get you up the scale a little.... What do you think you'd be able to eat?
C: A piece of fruit.
T: Sounds like a good start. When would you be able to eat that?
C: When the others are having their lunch.
T: Would you eat it *with* your friends?
C: I suppose I could, yes.
T: What kind of fruit will you be eating?
C: Some grapes or an apple ...
T: What will that feel like?
C: I'll start to feel a bit more normal ... eating when they do.
T: That sounds a little bit like your Miracle Day, eating something with your friends.... How likely is it that, between now and when we next meet, you will be able to eat a piece of fruit? Say 0 is not at all likely, 10 is you definitely will do it ...
C: Very likely ... I'd think an 8 or 9.

It is important to get as much detail as possible from the client. The more simple, realistic and achievable the picture, the easier it will be to put it into practice. It is also a good idea to scale the client's determination/ability, e.g. by asking:

"How likely is it that between now and the next session you will have done (X, Y or Z)?"

or:

"So you are at a 6 now, what needs to happen to get you even more determined, say a 7?"

or:

"What will the next point on the scale look like?"

or:

"Who or what could help you to move up a point?"

Together, client and therapist devise achievable goals that will help the client move up the scale to a suitable point for therapy to finish. My clients often opt for 7 to 8. In order to know when this stage has been reached and it is time to stop, they are asked to describe in detail what life would look like then. Interestingly, clients who have perfectionist tendencies, often associated with anorexia nervosa, may go for 10 or even higher!

At times I have successfully challenged this:

T: So where do you need to get to on a scale of 0-10, for us to know that we

C: can stop working together?
C: Oh ... I think maybe 15!
T: Wow, *fifteen!* Scrape-me-off-the-ceiling time, then! [Laughter] How will people cope?
C: Hmm....Yes, always being at 15 would be a bit much, maybe!
T: So what do you think?
C: Uh ... 8 or 9?
T: So what will you be doing at 8 or 9?

Challenging the client's ideal point worked in the example above, but I have learned not to question it as a matter of course: if it appears that the client gets some sense of security from thinking their recovery must be (more than) perfect, then this needs to be respected. Trying to get them to be satisfied with a lower point on the scale would be a "solution-forced" approach. I have found that most clients mellow after a few sessions and getting to 7 or 8 becomes "good-enough". Very few of my clients finish therapy at 10.

Exceptions

Throughout the course of the work, the therapist will be on the look out for exceptions – the times the problem is not there, or the client is better able to cope. Clients are often unaware of what they are already achieving and are pleasantly surprised when the therapist presents them with factual evidence. Exceptions can be found in the client's story, the Miracle Day description, or by asking a direct question, e.g. "Are there times the problem is slightly less?" Alternatively, the therapist can re-frame what a client has just said:

C: There's hardly a time that I'm not bingeing.
T: There are times that you do not binge. [Followed by: "What do you do instead?"]

Mary (25) came to see me for support to overcome anorexia with bulimic tendencies. The illness had caused her to give up her job and she had moved back to the parental home. As far as she was concerned her life was black and bleak: "I can't do *anything* anymore, I have *no* confidence!" Her Miracle Day went as follows:

M: I will be able to get up and feel refreshed. I'll have some breakfast without feeling guilty. I will have moved back with my friends and have a job. I'll go out with my friend to a café and have a cappuccino and a cake, and we will go shopping and have fun. We'll be able to have lunch together. In the afternoon I will do some painting, and in the evening we go out to a night-club.

I'll feel confident, able to start up conversations. People will see me smiling and interacting ...

I asked her if tiny bits of the miracle were already happening and after a long pause she said this:
M: I did go to a café with a friend yesterday, and although I didn't eat a cake, I was able to have a coffee! And I did enjoy myself! I know I'm not earning money at the moment, because I'm not well enough to do a full-time job, but I'm applying to do some volunteer work. I haven't been able to go to a pub or a club with my friend yet, but I visited a friend at her home the other day.
This showed Mary that she was already making significant changes, and she recognised that when these small parts of the miracle were occurring, the eating disorder took a back seat and she felt better about herself. On the strength of this she was able to set herself some achievable goals that would help her get higher up the scale.

Small, achievable steps
Often, clients enter therapy because previous attempts at recovery have not been successful. This could be because the goals that were set (personally or by a professional) did not meet their needs. And now they have put themselves in another vulnerable position by opening up to the possibility of change. What a courageous thing to do!

The eating disorder has been a security blanket and although it has become dirty and smelly, it may still provide a degree of comfort and is thus worth clinging onto. Some professionals assume that clients can just ditch the eating disorder by "eating normally" and encourage them to do so against all the odds. This will be perceived as whipping away the security blanket, and is not only cruel and abusive but serves to make a clients feel inadequate and a failure. It will have an adverse effect on recovery.

The first thing clients want to find out is if they can trust the therapist. Anxious thoughts may spin around their heads: " Will she understand and support me? Will she push me too hard and will I be able to live up to her expectations?"

So what does the client need in order to feel safe, secure and supported? I think appropriate goal-setting is paramount, and the solution-focused therapist comes alongside the client, ensuring that the pace of therapy is matched with the speed the client is willing and able to travel. To give clients a sense of accomplishment, great attention is given to making the goals attainable. This process is facilitated by working in small, achievable steps.

Annie (25) suffered from anorexia nervosa and was discharged from a specialist clinic having regained her weight, but no therapeutic follow-up support had been provided. Eventually she was referred to me via the Community Mental Health Team because she had started reducing her food intake.

Her Miracle Day showed her living independently, returned to her teaching job, being able to eat without feeling guilty and having an active social life. She was, however, extremely ambivalent about "getting better" because to her this was synonymous with putting on vast amounts of weight.

At the start of therapy she was at 2-3 on the scale. Feeling low and depressed, she had stopped eating at lunch time four days per week, but was still able to eat lunch on the remaining three days. Her aim was to get to 8. By the third session she had progressed to 5. For many years she had been stuck in her problem, mourning what the eating disorder had stolen from her. But solution-focused therapy had made her look towards the future, and to what she really wanted from life. It had given her hope and she had started to make some small changes. What needed to happen next was to find out what else she needed to do to reach 8. We worked with small, achievable steps to support her as she her increased her food intake, and we looked at other benefits of getting better.

A: [At 5…] I am beginning to worry a bit less about maybe having to have a bigger dress size. I'm beginning to accept that being underweight is not making me feel happy … so I'd like to start eating lunch one extra day per week, but I'm too scared to do it.

T: OK…. Can you tell me what would be the benefit of eating one more lunch per week?

A: I know that if I eat properly it will give me energy. I need to eat some more so I can start doing things again

T: What would it enable you to do?

A: Go out more … live a little! Get my sense of humour back, be more optimistic …

T: Hmm, I see…. So to achieve that, as you say, you need to eat more. Now, we already know that you *can* have lunch, because you do so 3 days per week, which is great. Say you are able to have lunch on "day 4." Where will that get you on your scale?

A: I think it would get me to 6.

T: How likely is it that you will have some lunch on day 4 between now and the next session?

A: Not very likely… I'd say a 2 or 3.

T: It's great that you are even *contemplating* the idea of eating some more … but actually *achieving* it is a bit more tricky?

A: Yes.
T: I wonder, what is your eating disorder telling you to eat on that fourth day?
A: I dunno ... something big and fattening ... that's the scary part, you see!
T: Fish and chips and bread'n'butter pudding with custard for afters?
A: [Laughter] Yeah, something like that!
T: So.... On a scale of 0-10, where at 0 there's not a snowball's chance in hell and at 10 you'd eat fish, chips and pud' for definite ...
A: [Laughter] Yes, that would be a 0.
T: [Dryly] OK ... so we won't be tempted to try that then. [Laughter] I'm curious though.... What do you eat on the other 3 days?
A: Something healthy ... baked potato and salad, pasta, a vegetarian meal.
T: So you know how to look after yourself then. You'd consider these "safe" meals?
A: Yes.
T: And on our scale, how likely would it be that you'd eat one of those "safe" meals on the fourth day? Zero is not at all, 10 is for certain.
A: I should think about 5.
T: So we're getting closer. Now.... For just *one extra day*, what will you *definitely* be able to eat between now and the next session?
A: [Thinks for a while] I think ... I can eat a piece of toast.
T: This is for definite?
A: Yes. I can do that.
T: So where would you scale that? Zero is no chance, 10 definite.
A: A 10.
T: A 10! That sounds great! You are convinced that between now and when we next meet, you will have a piece of toast on day 4 instead of having nothing at all.
A: Yes.
T: Now, I wonder if you could carefully notice what difference that makes to you. Does eating this piece of toast on day 4 make you feel better? You said, more energy, more positive, more confidence
A: Yes.
T: Does it take you a bit higher than the 5 where you are now, maybe to a 5.1? And if it does make you feel better, could you try it again on another day?
A: Maybe ...
T: But if it makes you feel worse, we have to think of another option.... Does that seem OK?
A: Yes, that will be OK. I will do it for one day for definite, and then decide if I want to have a piece of toast on another day.

Annie's example shows a variety of interventions and attitudes commonly found in solution-focused sessions: compliments, exceptions, small steps, scales, affirmations, curiosity, awareness of the client's boundaries, limitations and capabilities. But above all a deep respect for the client.

This way of questioning led Annie from anxiously contemplating a huge leap (I guess she'd need to get nearer to 10 to eat fish and chips!) to making a definite commitment to eat toast, and we identified the benefits this would bring. Initially, she thought she had to jump from a 5 to a 6 but we broke it down to a manageable step: from 5 to 5.1. And on the strength of that she would consider trying to eat some toast on another day as well.

This is referred to as "leading from behind". The therapist knows that the eating disorder is "out to get the client", and the quickest way to make a client fail and feel useless is to set the goals too high. Clients are usually hugely relieved when they realise the therapist is on their side and is prepared to work within the parameters of their abilities.

However well-matched a goal may appear within a session, clients may report having been unable to attain what they set out to do. This is normalised, and little time is given to exploring in detail why and how it went wrong. We work on de Shazer's premise: "If it doesn't work, stop doing it" (de Shazer, 1988). And, having learned from the mistake, a new and better goal is designed. Conversely, if it *has* worked, the client is encouraged to do more of it, or to use success as a springboard for the next step.

Break

Although it is not an essential part of solution-focused therapy, some therapists take a break before the end of the session to discuss the work with a colleague, or to gather their thoughts. This might mean leaving the room, or if that is not practical, asking the client's permission to have a few moments silence to reflect on what has been said and to formulate feedback. This feedback consists of sensitive compliments and, if appropriate, a collaboratively designed task is set.

Compliments

It is beneficial to end sessions on an upbeat note (Berg, 1993) and with a sense of having accomplished something. The therapist compliments the client on his or her strengths, coping strategies and any positive ways the problem is already being dealt with.

Task

A "homework task" is co-constructed. Left to their own devices, my clients often give themselves "mammoth" tasks. For example, a client who vomits after every meal might say, "Between now and when we next meet, I won't vomit at all!"

This stems from the perfectionist streak that many people in eating distress share. It is either all or nothing, so they must stop vomiting all together, or carry on as usual. Unfortunately the tasks they devise for themselves are often unachievable and they set themselves up to fail. Failure leads to more opportunities to "beat themselves up", thus lowering self-esteem and being further entrapped by the illness. So it is very important that tasks are easily achievable. And if the client is able to carry them out successfully once, they may decide try and do more of what works.

In the case of the person who wants completely to stop vomiting, the therapist could scale how convinced is the client that there will definitely be no vomiting between sessions. If the client still on being right at the top, then the task is agreed upon. However, most clients will recognise that this is quite unlikely to happen, so a more realistic mission could be a "noticing task", such as "Between now and when we next meet, I will make a mental note of the times I do not vomit after a meal. What do I do instead? How does it make me feel?"

The task is discussed in the next session, and if it was carried out successfully the client could try to do some more of what worked. If not, a new, more appropriate task could be constructed.

Follow-up appointments

Each subsequent session starts with, "What has been good since we last met?" This is a very directional question which shows the therapist's confidence that clients have the ability to turn life around independent of therapy.

Sometimes clients report, "Nothing good has happened at all." However, as they share how awful things have been, they invariably come up with a wealth of positive incidents and coping strategies. But it seems as if the eating disorder has successfully blocked these from their view. I really enjoy picking up on these exceptions, and feeding them back. Clients can visibly change from despondency to optimism.

Occasionally they are not able to see anything positive at all. In this case the therapist can ask, "How come it has not got any worse?" which re-focuses on the client's competence that at least something is occurring that prevents them slipping further.

2.

WHAT ARE EATING DISORDERS?

> The nosology of insanity, the etiology, the symptomatology, pathology, diagnosis, prognosis, the care - how nicely the textbooks classify everything! How accurately they defined the idiot, the cretin, the imbecile, the epileptic, the hysteric, hypochondriac, and neurasthenic. Instead of admitting that little was known about what went on in the human brain, either healthy or sick, the professors stacked up Latin names.
>
> From The Estate, Isaac Bashevis Singer,
> (found in Abraham and Llewellyn-Jones, 1984)

Labels and diagnoses

I avoid the use of labels and "pathologising terms" such as "She is an anorexic," because they can be difficult to shed. Instead, I prefer to say "She is recovering from anorexia," which adds a positive note, separates the illness from the person and allows client and therapist to form an alliance against the problem.

The philosopher Michel Foucault showed how seemingly neutral medical diagnoses were in fact "weapons of power", facilitating the use of force on "deviants" in order to make them "normal" (Foucault, 1973; Rabinow, 1984). I think diagnoses must be made with utmost care as diagnostic categorisation is generally negative. For some people a diagnosis confirms the existence of a disease and the need to see a doctor for a prescription. Diagnoses can inhibit therapy through stigmatisation, or as many of my clients have experienced, can slow recovery through generalisation and stereotyping, with attitudes such as, "Oh, she's got an eating disorder, therefore she is manipulative/an impossible case/resistant."

Having said all this, there are instances where giving a diagnosis can be therapeutic. Some clients want to put a name to their condition, because "knowing the enemy" enables them to fight against it.

Expertise
Underlying issues and causation are not dwelt on within the solution-focused therapy session. Therefore, being an expert in eating disorders or indeed in any specialist field is not essential. However, Palmer and Treasure (1999) state that eating disorders have difficult psychological and physical aspects, and if services are to be optimal, neither can be neglected. I think that, although not necessarily explored with clients within sessions, a reasonable understanding of psychological, psychosocial, physical and physiological changes inherent in eating disorders is important both to ensure safe and appropriate treatment, and to aid communication within multi-disciplinary teams.[†] Indeed, therapists working predominantly in this field will inevitably gain considerable knowledge. One outcome of my research was that the participants perceived this as helpful. When I ask if clients have noticed any "pre-session change" I am frequently told, "The thought of coming to see an expert gave me hope, which helped me to start making some changes."

So, in support of good practice, this chapter describes briefly what is generally understood by the term "eating disorders". The main conditions are anorexia nervosa, bulimia nervosa and compulsive binge-eating disorder. Other, more recently described difficulties are compulsive dieting, athletica nervosa and unspecified eating disorders.

Clients who have a combination of these can display co-morbid symptoms, such as infertility, osteoporosis, drug or alcohol abuse, and/or psychological disorders such as depression, self-harm (e.g. cutting), suicidal ideas, or obsessive-compulsive habits. The problem profile can vary significantly over time; in different phases of the illness, anorexia nervosa, bulimia nervosa, binge-eating or personality disorder could all be diagnosed (Robinson, 1998). In other words, clients can drift in and out of these disorders, perhaps from anorexia to bulimia, to compulsive binge eating and back again.

Body mass index.
Weight is an important aspect of any eating disorder and the body mass index (BMI) can be calculated to establish if a person is under-, over-, or at normal weight.

$$BMI = \frac{\text{weight in kilograms}}{\text{height in meters} \times \text{height in meters}}$$

The outcome is interpreted as follows:
 -16: Extremely underweight
 16-18: Significantly underweight

---

† A comprehensive description of the psychological and physiological complications of eating disorders can be found in European Eating Disorders Review, 2000, Wiley & Sons, Baffins Lane, Chichester, West Sussex PO19 1UD, UK.

20-25: Healthy weight
27-30: Overweight
30-40: Significantly overweight
40+: Extremely overweight

As with all calculations this is a rule of thumb only, and must never be used as a single diagnosing factor. The psychological distress is of equal importance, and clients can be suffering to a dangerous degree even if the BMI is not significantly low or high.

Anorexia nervosa
This condition has been medically recognised for over a century and affects mainly females, but is rising in the male population. Onset is generally thought to be early adolescence (Bruch, 1974, 1978), but it is increasingly found in younger children and in the elderly.

To diagnose anorexia nervosa[†], the following conditions must obtain:
- The person is significantly underweight as a result of his/her own efforts and the Body Mass Index is below 17.5.
- Females who should have menstrual periods (between the age of 12-55 approx.) report an absence of three consecutive menses.
- There is deep concern about body shape and intense fear of putting on weight. In spite of being underweight, many people suffering from anorexia nervosa regard themselves as fat.

The under eating in anorexia nervosa is often combined with activities such as laxative and/or diuretic abuse, self-induced vomiting and over-exercising, which can have the following psychological and physical effects:

Psychological effects of anorexia nervosa
- Anxiety
- Depression
- Feeling of obesity
- Social isolation.
- Mood swings
- Co-morbid psychiatric disorders, such as compulsive behaviour, self-mutilation, sexual promiscuity, kleptomania, etc.

Physical complications of anorexia nervosa
- Oral: erosion of the teeth due to regurgitated stomach acid.
- Gastro-intestinal: reduced muscle power of the bowel and stomach wall; peristalsis is reduced.

† DSM3 criteria, American Psychiatric Association, 1987.

- Gastric: reduced stomach size. Delayed stomach emptying causes abnormal feeling of fullness; client feels uncomfortably full/nauseous even after small amounts are eaten.
- Hepatic: resulting from (paracetamol) overdose or fatty infiltration of the liver.
- Colonic: constipation due to restricted food intake or damage to the bowel wall due to laxative abuse, resulting in faecal incontinence.
- Reproductive: Amenorrhoea in females, or menstrual irregularity. Infertility in males and females. (These dysfunctions are usually restored with weight recovery.)
- Dermatological: excessive hair growth (laguno, a downy type of hair covering the whole body). Dry skin, itching, and deregulation of body temperature; generally feeling cold and shivery; brittle nails and hair.
- Renal: impaired kidney function.
- Skeletal: osteoporosis. Between the age of 15 and 25, stores of calcium are laid down in the skeleton. If the body suffers malnourishment during this period, osteoporosis will occur, causing fractures and malformation. If the client recovers before the age of 25, reasonable replenishment of calcium stores can be achieved.
- Cardiovascular: structural changes of the heart, cardiac failure, re-feeding oedema, ECG abnormalities.
- Neurological: generalised muscle weakness, peripheral nerve dysfunction, loss of sense in toes and fingers.
- Biochemical/Endocrinological: electrolyte (hypokalaemia, hyponatraemia) and vitamin imbalance due to starvation or vomiting/laxative/diuretic abuse.
- Haematological: anaemia, abnormal white cell count, bone marrow changes
- Often chronic in nature, this condition has a mortality rate of around 20%, the highest associated for any psychiatric illness (Treasure, 1999). About half the deaths result from medical complications and the remainder are suicides.

Some typical ideas and thought patterns
I am fat. I am unhappy. If I were thinner I would be happier. What can I do to get thinner? How can I avoid eating today? Where can I secretly exercise? How can I work off/purge the food I have just eaten? I am getting thinner. This feels good. People are giving me compliments. They admire me. Feeling in control is good. I must be "good" (eat as little as possible). I must try not to be "bad" (eat something). Where can I hide the food I've just been given? How many calories are in that? If I eat that, I will put on masses of weight. If I eat that I won't be able to stop, so I'd better not eat at all. All my friends are thinner than me, so I'd better stay at home because they will be disgusted at my size. I don't have to eat, because I never feel hungry. Food does not taste nice anymore. I'm not good enough. I'm a failure. No

one loves me. No one cares. No one understands. People don't give me compliments anymore. They say I'm too thin, they are just jealous. I hate everyone. I hate myself. I'm a bad person. I don't deserve to eat anything. I'm hungry... no, I'm not hungry. I am lonely, I feel out of control.

A few common tell-tale signs

Clinically, loss of weight is main diagnostic factor of anorexia nervosa, but the illness must not be diagnosed on BMI alone. The food-focusing aspect may be apparent and troubling the client long before the BMI gets to danger level.

Many clients report specific behaviour. It is usual that, however emaciated they may be, they still consider themselves fat. They may weigh themselves several times a day, or undertake excessive exercise (jogging, gym workouts and swimming are fanatically pursued). Normal activities are turned into exercise (e.g. running up and down stairs four times instead of once). Low or no-fat foods are chosen. Large amounts of salt, herbs or spices to are added to food to enhance flavour which would have normally been brought out by the fat content. Unusual food combinations, such as sausages and marmalade, cheese and strawberry jam, are eaten. This is combined with an intense interest in food: preparing large amounts and feeding them to family and friends without touching any of it themselves, is normal. Anorexics may collect recipes, or seek jobs related to food. Ritualistic behaviour develops (e.g. cutting up food in certain ways, only eating things in groups of four, counting how many times a mouthful is chewed). They are often unable to eat when others are present. They know the calorific value of everything they eat, and of most things they do not eat, while considering certain foods to be "bad and sinful" and avoiding them. Anorexics drink tea and coffee to fill themselves up, and chew gum excessively. They become socially isolated, and lie about what has or has not been eaten. There are mood swings, and episodes of high activity followed by burnout.

Many people who suffer from anorexia nervosa say that they have either lost their appetite ("Food just doesn't taste nice anymore, it has lost its appeal"), or that they feel uncomfortably full or even nauseous after small amounts of food (e.g. a dry biscuit, a small banana).

In the event of a loss of taste, the taste-buds have temporarily "gone to sleep". But they can be re-activated by slowly introducing new tastes, as one would do with a baby.

In the case of satiation and nausea, it is due to the stomach size being reduced because of the lack of food that has been ingested over a period of time. Added to this, the muscles in the stomach wall have lost their tension. Therefore, the stomach is able to hold less and in addition will take longer to digest food. It is advisable to serve small, regular snacks to overcome this. Clients suffering in this way need specialist dietetic advice to recover their weight.

Bulimia nervosa
Mainly affecting Caucasian women, with an onset most commonly described in teenage, this condition was first mentioned in the mid-1970s in reports describing American college girls with "binge-purge syndrome" (Fairburn, 1995). The problem is now becoming more prevalent in young men who feel society's pressure to be lean and muscular.

Initially thought to be a variant of anorexia nervosa, it soon became clear that bulimia (eating like a bull) was a significant health problem in its own right. Symptoms observed in bulimia nervosa are:
- Recurrent episodes of binge eating (on average two binges per week for three months minimum) coupled with a sense of loss of control.
- Excessive concern about body shape and an intense fear of weight gain. A variety of extreme measures are used to control shape or weight, e.g. self-induced vomiting, laxative or diuretic abuse, over-exercising, and periods of dieting/fasting.
- The person is not significantly underweight (BMI typically between twenty and twenty-five).†

The psychological and physical effects of bulimia nervosa are similar to those experienced in anorexia nervosa:

Psychological effects of bulimia nervosa
- Anxiety
- Depression
- Feeling of obesity
- Social isolation
- Mood swings
- Co-morbid psychiatric disorders
- Feeling of loss of control and shame
- Secrecy: on the outside, sufferers can appear happy and competent. Their destructive behaviour may go undetected for many years because generally weight is within normal limits, but it can be an illness with fatal consequences.

Physical Complications of Bulimia Nervosa:
- Oral: erosion of the teeth due to regurgitated stomach acid. Swelling of salivary glands ("hamster face").
- Oesophageal: the action of vomiting increases pressure on the delicate blood vessels in the oesophageal wall, causing varicose veins. This may result in ruptured oesophageal varices (blood in vomit).

† DSM3 criteria, American Psychiatric Association, 1987

- Gastro-intestinal: reduced motility, slowing down of peristalsis.
- Gastric: delayed stomach emptying and abnormal satiety level. Feeling uncomfortably full/nauseous after eating.
- Colonic: damage to the bowel wall due to laxative abuse, resulting in faecal
- Incontinence.
- Hepatic: resulting from (paracetamol) overdose or fatty infiltration of the liver
- Reproductive: females experience disturbed menses. Infertility occurs both in males and females, but is usually restored when nutrition is stabilised
- Dermatological: dry skin, itching, disregulation of body temperature and erosion of the fingers used to induce vomiting.
- Renal: impaired kidney function.
- Skeletal: osteoporosis (see anorexia nervosa).
- Cardiovascular: structural changes of the heart, cardiac failure, ECG abnormalities
- Biochemical/Endocrine: electrolyte (hypokalaemia, hyponatraemia) and vitamin imbalance due to starvation or vomiting/laxative/diuretic abuse.
- Haematological: anaemia and abnormal white cell count.

Some typical ideas and thought patterns
I am unhappy. This is because I'm fat. I am out of control. I might as well eat the whole lot. What can I do to lose weight? I have to "get rid of it". I am so disgusting, greedy, out of control. I will make myself sick after I've eaten. Will the loo flush properly? Will anyone hear me being sick? I need to lose more weight. I'll try laxatives. If I go to that chemist again they will rumble me, so I must find another one. When will the laxatives start to work? Will I be near a loo? Vomiting and laxatives alone are not doing the trick. I will need to exercise more. And more. I know I can stop the laxatives and vomiting if I want to. I won't do it yet though.... Today I will not binge-vomit at all.... Now I've broken my promise, I might as well carry on. I'm useless. I can't cope. If people knew what I am really like, they'd be disgusted. What a waste of food. I am so ashamed of myself. No one must know what I am up to. Where can I get hold of some more food? I can't stop binge-purging and exercising anymore. I feel out of control.

A few common tell-tale signs
Feeling fat and hoarding food. Evidence of laxatives (empty containers). Disappearing to lavatory straight after or even during meals. Excessive flushing and cleaning of the toilet. Damage to teeth. Swollen salivary glands – the "hamster face". Regular complaints of sore throats, constipation, feeling of obesity. Drinking a lot with meals to facilitate vomiting. Relentless exercising. Secrecy and lying about what they have or have not eaten. Boasting about what they can eat without putting on

weight. Intense interest in food, calories and cooking. Co-morbid symptoms such as sexual promiscuity or loss of libido, compulsive shopping, stealing and obsessive-compulsive habits. Mood swings. Feeling out of control around food: either eating too much or not at all. Social isolation.

People suffering from bulimia nervosa generally are of normal weight and appear to cope with life reasonably well.

Compulsive binge-eating

This condition came to light in the mid-1980s when it became evident that about a quarter of those seeking treatment for obesity had binge-eating problems. Obesity is a chronic disease, which results from an imbalance between energy intake and energy expenditure and is a complex combination of genetic and environmental factors. With binge eating, genuinely large amounts of food are consumed at one time, leaving the person feeling guilty, uncomfortable and depressed. Sufferers do not subject themselves to extreme weight control measures, so BMI is high.

The classifications are:

Overweight:	BMI >25	
Class 1 Obesity:	BMI >30	(moderate to increased health risk)
Class 2 Obesity:	BMI 35 to 39	(severely increased health risk)
Class 3 Obesity:	BMI >40	(very severe increased health risk)

Men and women ranging from age 20-50 are more evenly affected, while African-Americans are as much at risk as Caucasians (Fairburn, 1995).

Psychological effects of compulsive binge eating
- Anxiety
- Depression
- Feeling of fatness
- Social isolation
- Mood swings
- Co-morbid psychiatric disorders
- Feeling of loss of control and shame
- Secrecy (hoarding food, bingeing in private)
- Lethargy and fatigue

Physical complications of compulsive binge eating
- Oral: erosion of the teeth due to excessive intake of sugar-loaded foods and fizzy drinks.
- Gastric: uncomfortable feeling of fullness, ruptured stomach wall.
- Hormonal: pre-disposition to diabetes mellitus.
- Dermatological: stretch-marks, itching, perspiration, sores due to friction in

skin folds.
- Cardiovascular: structural changes of the heart, cardiac failure, high blood pressure, ECG abnormalities.
- Musculo-skeletal: over-stressed muscles and erosion of joints due to obesity.
- Increased mortality rate.

Some typical ideas and thought patterns
I'm unhappy. I'm fat. I'm disgusting. I'm useless. I will have some food to make me feel better. I will start a diet tomorrow and to prevent temptation, I will eat all the cakes and biscuits in the house today. I didn't start my diet. I am a failure. I'll eat something to make myself feel better and will start dieting tomorrow. I feel fat, I feel uncomfortable. I am never satisfied. Why did I do it? I have no self-control. People look at me with disgust. I don't want to go out. I can't get clothes to fit me … this is upsetting. I will eat something to make me feel better. When I eat I can forget about my unhappiness. Why can't I control what I eat? Tomorrow I will be "good". I've messed up again. I will be happy when I'm thinner. I will lose a stone in a month. I will start the x/y/z diet.… I have not been able to stick to the diet. Failed again … eat some more.

Tell-tale signs
Obesity. Eating genuinely large quantities of food and secretly eating even more (evidenced by discarded containers and wrappers). Happy on the outside, but miserable within. Unable to resist food. Self-consciousness. "Being good" in public, then bingeing when alone. Amnesia regarding what has actually been consumed during the day.

Related Problems:

Compulsive ("Yo-Yo") dieting
Dieting is a behaviour indicator of body dissatisfaction. This is supported by the dominant discourse of today, where being thin equals being happy, fit, healthy, successful, elegant, self-possessed etc. Women in particular are encouraged to be below their "set point" weight,[†] although the pressure on men to possess a "six-pack" is ever-increasing, and places similar pressures on them to try and alter body shape through diet and/or exercise.

But dieting is still most common among women; most sources state that about 25% of men diet at some time in life, compared to 95% women (only 2% of Weight Watchers are men). In general, men diet because they want to be healthy, women because they want to increase self-esteem.

---

† Genetically pre-set weight does not always tally with what western society dictates women (and increasingly men) "should" look like.

Only 5% of non-obese dieters report sustained weight loss (Grogan, 1999). The rest regains the weight, which leads to a sense of failure and low self-esteem. A vicious circle manifests itself. As thin equals happy, healthy and attractive, then weight needs to be lost in order to feel better. As soon as the diet stops, the weight is re-gained; a new diet is started, weight is lost and then re-gained. Yo-yo dieting takes a hold, resulting in ever-sinking self-esteem. To make matters worse, dieting induces physiological changes such as a lowered metabolic rate, which will make future weight loss more difficult.

Some typical ideas and thought patterns
Everyone around me is thinner than I am. They are happy and healthy. I am unhappy so I'll go on a diet. I lose some weight and feel a bit better about myself. I've reached my target. I'll stop the diet. Oh no, I'm putting on weight again! It's all gone back on … I don't fit in my new clothes anymore … better go on another diet.

Athletica nervosa
Moderate exercise improves health and produces endorphins, the hormones that generate a "feel-good factor". However, if exercising is taken to the extreme, and develops into a compulsive activity, it increases body dissatisfaction and sufferers will try to get a grip on their lives through controlling their shape in a way that is akin to, or may develop into, food restriction and full-blown anorexia nervosa. In fact, this is considered a variant of anorexia nervosa and as such is treated in a similar way. The psychological distress connected with athletica nervosa is similar to the above disorders, while the physical consequences are due to over-stressing the musculo-skeletal system.

Some typical ideas and thought patterns
Exercise is good for me. Look at me, I am lean and strong. This feels good. People are giving me compliments. I must do some more. I could start exercising several times each day instead of just once. When I exercise I don't worry. Everyone else is still in bed but I'm out jogging at 5.30 in the morning. I feel virtuous. Then I'll go to the gym and beat the hell out of the instruments. I'm trying to be the fittest and strongest. Others admire my lean body, fitness and willpower. I feel a little tired. No I don't, I'll exercise some more. If anyone puts themselves between me and my training regime I'll bite their heads off. I feel irritable. I'll go for a jog as it blots out my thoughts. I'm beginning to ache…. Do I have to get up at 5 again? I feel out of control….

Unspecified Eating Disorders
In addition to the above well-documented disorders, there is a group of unspecified difficulties, e.g.

Night bingeing: sufferers cope well during the day (although they are often found to under-nourish themselves in the daytime) but are restless and wakeful in the night, subjecting themselves to secretive, solitary episodes of eating while others are asleep.

Selective ("fussy") eating: there is a very strict protocol of what can and cannot be eaten. These clients tend to run into difficulties when the chosen food is out of season or unavailable, and a new, "safe" food has to be chosen.

Chewing/Spitting: people afflicted by this condition are generally able to put a wide variety of food into their mouth, but are unable to swallow "dangerous" foods, in particular those high in fat and refined sugars.

Difficulty chewing/swallowing solid foods: related to chew/spitting, it may be difficult to put solid food in the mouth and often these clients exist on a liquid diet.

Orthorexia: a new term, meaning an *unhealthy* pre-occupation with *healthy* foods. Clients will only eat "health foods", are often vegetarian or vegan, or will only eat low fat and low sugar content meals, etc. They *never* allow themselves to relax the rules (e.g. joining friends in a fry-up) The rules of healthy eating become more rigid and this restriction has a negative influence on the overall quality of life.

All these conditions have destructive, potentially fatal, consequences. The psychological difficulty of this client group is similar to the other eating disorders. Food is regarded as problematic and much time that could be better spent elsewhere is wasted on considering calorific value, fat and sugar content of food, potential weight gain or loss, and so on.

Physiologically, clients may suffer malnutrition resulting in any or all of the side effects described above.

Coping Strategy

I have come to regard eating disorders as a client's unique way of coping with stress, anxiety and difficult or hurtful situations, because:
- When attention is focused around food, it obliterates the underlying distress.
- If there is a low sense of self-esteem, the feeling of "control" as seen in anorexia nervosa, athletica nervosa, selective eating or dieting, can induce a sense of triumph, power and success.
- In compulsive binge eating and bulimia nervosa, the binge provides a temporary "out-of-body experience", soothing the sufferer for a short while by hiding the problem.
- The "emptying" caused by vomiting or laxative abuse can be experienced as a cleansing action to purge the sufferer of bad feelings.

We know that food focus can successfully mask underlying stress and anxiety. Initially, it brings a sense of control or comfort, but this is shallow and as time passes the emerging eating disorder starts to assert itself. When the coping strategy becomes less attractive or effective the sufferer may seek help, or referral for treatment is made by a health professional, friend or relative. In my practice, I try to form a collaborative relationship with the client and we challenge the usefulness of destructive coping strategies while other, self-nurturing ways of coping are amplified or constructed.

Disordered eating

Fairburn (1995) suggests that all eating disorders are a form of "binge eating". The client with anorexia nervosa has "subjective binges": normal, or even tiny amounts of food are considered a binge and have to be disposed of by exercising or purge methods, or compensated for by a period of starvation.

Those suffering from bulimia or compulsive binge eating indulge in "objective binges", where seriously large amounts of food are consumed.

Compared to overcoming other afflictions (we can stay alive without drugs, we do not need nicotine to survive, and can sustain life by drinking water rather than alcohol), recovery from eating distress is complex. To the client with eating difficulties, food is a wolf in sheep's clothing. Living beings need food, yet food is also the enemy – there is no escape. Not only do sufferers need to overcome the stresses that led to the eating disorder in the first place, they also have to work on a change of lifestyle in terms of nutrition.

Causes and reasons

Sometimes clients come to therapy to learn *why* they have an eating disorder. No one has yet found a simple answer and on the premise that we do not need to know where we have come from in order to know where we are heading, solution-focused therapists avoid spending time trying to find the answer to the 'Why?' question. What may be of interest is the client's answer to questions such as these:

"Suppose we found an answer, what difference would that make?"

"Imagine you discovered the cause, what would that enable you to achieve?"

or

"Let's pretend you have the answer. Now what can you do?"

I become openly and unashamedly directional when clients are stuck in the "Why" question. I invite them to start working in a solution-focused way, promising that if it doesn't work, they can bring their spade for problem-digging to the next session. Most clients forget that they came wanting answers in the first place, or if they do remember, they agree that "knowing why" is not necessary in order to make progress.

If "Why?" continues to be an issue, I simply explain that no one cause is yet identified and that their eating disorder could be due to any of the reasons given below. If they are still not satisfied, I explain that I do not work in a problem-focused way and refer them to a therapist who does.

Although solution-focused therapy does not dwell on causes, it is important for the therapist to have a global idea of underlying and contributory factors in order to provide a safe service and to facilitate communication with other health professionals. It is understood that a fusion of multiple aspects is likely to lead to the development of an eating disorder. These are most commonly thought to be the following:

Psychological
- Parent-child relationships
- Anxiety around growing up and the maturation process, particularly relating to taking on adult responsibilities
- Sexual abuse
- Depression in childhood and/or adulthood
- Low self-esteem, lack of confidence
- Addictive or compulsive behaviour in the family
- Bullying/peer pressure
- Intense school/work-related stress
- Perfectionism
- Grieving process reaction
- Sibling rivalry

Physical
- Anxiety around growing up and the maturation process, particularly related to change of body shape
- Food intolerance/allergies
- Research is currently being undertaken to find genetic origins (Hepworth, 1999; Gilbert, 2000).

Social
- Giving undue importance to weight and shape
- Measuring success and happiness in kilograms
- Copycat behaviour (particularly bulimia nervosa)

Dieting
As mentioned earlier, eating disorders often follow a period of dieting. Fuelled by guilt and negative thought patterns, there is a complex and dynamic relationship between dieting and body dissatisfaction (Grogan, 1999; Warde, 1997). When diets fail, feelings of lack of control and lowered self-esteem ensue. Some sense of control can be regained by anorexic or bulimic behaviour, or the pain is dulled momentarily by

"comfort eating". Dieting can have negative implications both physiologically and psychologically.

Physiologically, the metabolic rate is upset by the pattern of restrictive episodes followed by binge eating: the body becomes more adept at conserving energy in order to cope with the next bout of starvation. Pulse and blood pressure decrease, limbs grow colder, energy level drops and consequently it becomes harder to lose weight.

Psychologically, eating disorders of the restrictive type (anorexia nervosa, bulimia nervosa, excluding specific foods) can have their origin in diet episodes. Women in particular tend to link being slim with being happy. They lose weight but don't feel any happier, so goalposts are moved and further weight is lost. Eventually they may discover that happiness is not obtainable in this way. Therapy supports them in achieving an acceptable lifestyle using strategies other than weight loss.

Media

Alongside this, media pressure cannot be overlooked; Rubenesque figures are not depicted favourably in the twenty-first century. Unfortunately, we have a genetically pre-set weight that does not tally with what western society dictates women "should" look like. So people diet in an attempt to conform to society's demands.

"Land of milk and honey" syndrome

Further tension arises between the opulence of food in the western world and the dominant discourse of today (slim equals healthy, attractive, successful and self-possessed). To compensate, people resort to slimming potions and lotions, lipo-suction and plastic surgery.

Evolution

Homo sapiens evolved gradually over six million years. Recently, we have "morphed" from nomadic hunter-gatherers into beings that place ready-made, microwaved meals on the table. But even until the mid-1950s, the choice of foods available was such that calorific intake and output were easily balanced: people burnt off what they ate. There was little, in comparison with today, available to nibble or graze on through the day, and in the scheme of things, obesity was relatively rare. Food was made out of complex ingredients, and bodies were tuned to cope with this.

But in the past fifty years technology has perfected refining and saturation techniques. Unbeknown to most people, our palates have been changed in the last few decades. Fast foods and ready-made meals have increased our appetite for highly refined, sugary foods to graze and snack on throughout the day.

This marked change in nutrition has been so rapid that our digestive system has not had time to adapt: ingesting high concentrations of refined carbohydrates and fat does not provide the measured release of energy we need to function at the optimum. As a result, we may feel sluggish and lethargic. In other words, our bodies are not tuned effectively to burn the fuel we put in.

Meanwhile, our lifestyle has become more sedentary with the increased use of automobiles, household appliances, television and computers. Statistics show that in the last twenty years the average person in Britain has become bigger, less physically active (children in particular), and more prone to heart disease, digestive troubles and strokes – although at the same time, as illustrated earlier, the dominant discourse in society increasingly dictates that we should be unnaturally thin!

Even our use of language has changed. What was once considered "good food" is now called "wicked" (or unhealthy), and what was once a treat is now a sin. Confusion abounds and eating disorders erupt.

3.

THE TREATMENT

Therapeutic support for people in eating distress: investigating what works

The prevalence of eating disorders, particularly in western society, means that it has become a topical subject for the media and more openly discussed than ever before. In England, the dramatic increase of reported eating distress[†] has led to the need for treatment being mentioned in the National Mental Health Framework Document (1999), but no effective protocol has been implemented and if treatment is available, it often leaves a lot to be desired. People in eating distress can feel ill-understood, particularly by health professionals.[*]

This situation seems to be common in other countries, too. The sad implication is that, even though someone may identify they have a problem, appropriate help is rarely available. If left untreated or undetected, eating disorders can lead to long-term problems with severe associated health risks.

Therapeutic options

Placing solution-focused therapy within therapeutic paradigms, McFarland (1995) observes four waves in the treatment of eating disorders. The first wave came early in the 20th century with the psycho-dynamic/analytic approach. This was followed by cognitive behavioural therapy, systemic therapy, and finally, in the 1980s, solution-focused therapy. They are all are in use today. While the first three therapeutic models tend to focus more on deficiency, the origins and maintenance of the problem (fatalistic approach), solution-focused therapy is different in that it looks away from the problem and towards the client's preferred future (optimistic approach). Although each group researches its own efficacy, there is not yet a globally accepted treatment for every disorder.

[†] 60.000 people diagnosed, actual number needing treatment likely to be in excess of 1 million – EDA,2000

[*] Eating Disorders Association paper: Eating Disorders, the needs for 2000 and beyond

I have worked with the solution-focused model since 1997 and decided to investigate my client's response to the methods and interventions specific to it, by making solution-focused therapy the qualitative research topic for my Masters dissertation. The research participants felt solution-focused therapy had a significant place in their recovery and I combined these findings with three years of follow-up details from my practice. The outcome of this exercise was very positive: 95% of clients were satisfied with their treatment and had made progress. The majority of these continued to make progress after therapy had finished. Clients indicated that the tools they had acquired in therapy helped them in this process.

Although my small inquiry cannot be considered as truly representative of the experience of all people recovering from eating disorders, I think it is fair to assume that others too might respond favourably to the solution-focused approach.

Another finding of my study was that not only does solution-focused therapy benefit many clients, it can also prevent burnout in the therapist. This appeared to be due to the fact that focusing on strengths and positive outcomes is less draining than accompanying the client into a slough of despondency.

I appreciate that not everyone will take to solution-focused therapy: some clients will prefer an analytic, psychodynamic approach, while others favour non-directive, person-centred therapy or the structure of cognitive behavioural work. Whatever the model, as Beales and Dolton (2000) say, "Therapy should be open and collaborative, giving maximum autonomy and responsibility for eating and other behaviour to the patient." The solution-focused approach also facilitates the swift development of a working alliance and offers the sense of hope they have lacked.

Therapeutic alliance
It is said that the theory which underpins therapy is less important than the relationship between client and therapist (Miller et al., 1997). It is now widely accepted that a good working relationship is facilitated by the core qualities of the therapist and mutual trust, so it is important to consider the fit between client and therapist. I think a good outcome is the result of model and therapist gelling with the needs and aims of the client. I have a conviction that my clients can get better, and feel strongly that no one deserves to have their lives, or the lives of those around them, ruined by eating distress. I think my personal philosophy and therapeutic stance have been greatly enhanced by the strength-based, positive attitudes fostered by solution-focused therapy.

What is recovery?
Some clients will have overcome their problem by the time therapy is finished, while others choose to terminate at a "good-enough" stage. In my experience, those in the latter group generally continue to make improvements after therapy has finished. I do

not have fixed ideas on what "recovery" looks like, because clients' needs are varied. Before embarking upon any treatment I think it is important to establish what the individual wants to achieve in terms of recovery, and what can realistically be accomplished within the allotted time or budget.

The concept of recovery varies from client to client. For some, it is acceptable to reduce binge-vomiting from several times per day to once weekly, where for others it might mean never binge-vomiting again. My task is to help clients reach the goal they have set themselves, provided it is within healthy limits.

The road to recovery is hazardous, and life is risky. However far clients may have come, they may find themselves reverting to old coping strategies when they are under pressure. This is normalised in the therapeutic process. Clients learn that with every slip they make, new strategies are taken on board that can help prevent them sliding quite so far the next time, as the following sequence of events shows.

Paul started his recovery at a point when he considered himself being at his lowest. He put himself as far down as 0 on the scale. Things were as bad as they had ever been. Life had become so unpleasant and intolerable that he considered ending it all. Yet there was still a small spark and he had just enough strength to do something to climb out of the pit. Somehow, he made a small change that got him to a 0.5. He was going along quite nicely, even got up to a 1 … until he met a point of stress and anxiety which forced him back into the pit. Shocked and bruised, he stayed there for a while, but picked himself up, dusted himself down and started climbing out again, this time as high as 1.5. Inevitably another event came along to push him down. But this time he managed to hang on at 0.5, and then he did not stay down as long as before. And as he picked himself up, he moved a little higher on the scale. Over time, new coping strategies, either self-made or co-constructed in therapy, helped him to inch to 3 or 4. And when he stumbled on the next patch of trouble he slipped to 2. This was an easier place to crawl up from, and having experienced the benefits of being 3 or 4, there was motivation to improve the situation quite quickly. And so he continued to set out markers along the way. He began to be able to say, "Today I feel at a 5 because I only vomited once. If I get to 6 I'll be vomiting only once per week, so what do I need to do to get there?"

For some clients this process can develop in a matter of weeks, while others take years of painful slipping and standing back up. But with the benefit of hindsight a steady progress can be detected in most cases.

Assessment

The first thing we need to know is this: What is it that the client wants to change? It seems straightforward enough to assume someone attends therapy to improve his or her circumstances. But with eating disorders this assumption can be fraught with difficulties, because although a client may well want to recover, there is often also a great need to hang on to the behaviours that, however destructive they may seem to others, have until now promised a degree of safety. For instance, someone suffering from bulimia nervosa may want to stop binge-vomiting, but not at the price of potentially piling on weight. In order to overcome this ambivalence, client and therapist map out what the client wants to change and how she will go about this in small, achievable steps. The exciting turning point is when the client begins to understand that she can change her "yes, but" situation ("Yes, I want to give up binge-vomiting, but I don't want to get fat") into a "yes, and" one ("Yes, I can lose weight, and give up binge-vomiting").

Scaling questions are invaluable in assessing not only where clients are and where they wish to get to, but also their determination and the likelihood that they will indeed bring about the necessary changes. This information can then be used to tailor the therapy to a client's individual needs.

The practitioner will assess whether a client would benefit from therapy, and if so, whether the work can be carried out in isolation, or whether it would be preferable to enlist the help of another health professional.

Clients will present for therapy with different needs, and to ensure safe and ethical practice it is important to have an awareness of what goes on at psychological, physical and physiological level. The lists of difficulties associated with eating distress mentioned in the previous chapter give an idea of what to look out for.

If there is any uncertainty about a client's well-being or concern about health aspects, it is *essential* to ask for help, e.g. from a doctor, nutritionist, community psychiatric nurse or the Eating Disorders Association.† Alternatively the therapist can encourage the client to ask for additional support.

I never conduct an assessment based on complicated forms and protocols, because they can be clinical and impersonal. I never weigh clients. If they do not mention their weight voluntarily (which most of them do anyway), and if it seems relevant to the work we do, I might casually refer to it in conversation. If I become worried about weight loss or gain, we devise an acceptable way to have this checked, e.g. by a practice nurse who will send me the relevant information. The things to look out for are body shape (signs of emaciation or clinical obesity) and any other visible signs of eating distress (see Chapter 2). Other specific information to assess the extent of a client's problem is gathered in "problem-free talk" and "problem definition". It is then that I pick up important pointers, such as a client's ways of controlling body shape and the extent of food-focusing. I will listen out for co-morbid symptoms (e.g. self-harm, alcohol abuse) and ask if a client is using medication or receiving other treatment. I am also interested to know if a client has received therapy before, and if so, what was helpful. Most clients also freely share what was *not* helpful, which tells me how not to go about things!

---

† details on p. 151

I divide clients' needs into eight groups and it goes without saying that these are generalisations and guidelines only.
- Clients may not need therapy because the support system they have in place (family and friends) is sufficient to promote recovery.
- Clients may need support from a therapist.
- Clients may benefit from therapy combined with medication or nutritional advice.
- Clients may need therapeutic, medical and nutritional support, and regular weight monitoring.
- Clients may require therapy, medication, nutritional counselling, weight monitoring and psychiatric help.
- Clients may be so severely ill that therapy is contra-indicated
- Clients may choose not to engage in the therapeutic process.
- Clients may have chronic problems.

Group 1
This could be called "Single-Session Therapy". It is clear that these clients are well motivated, the eating disorders not severe, and the support structure strong enough that further therapy is not necessary. All the clients need is to be nudged onto the right track. The useful coping strategies that are already in place are amplified, compliments are given, and therapy can finish with the assurance that a client can come back for a top-up session should this be necessary.

Group 2
These clients will have a non life-threatening form of eating distress. Solution-focused therapy is sufficient to help them break away from their problem. They do not require medication or regular weighing and, as such, it is safe to work with them without the need for extra support. They appreciate there is a problem, are motivated to change, and the amount of sessions needed is generally low.

Group 3
Clients often already take medication such as anti-depressants when they start therapy, and this can be of great support to them. The GP is in charge of the medication and oversees the general progress while therapy takes its normal course. If necessary, the help of a nutritionist may be sought to give expert advice on the "food side" of recovery and monitor weight, while the therapist concentrates on the psychological aspects. For many clients it is a relief not to have to talk about food and weight in therapy.

There may be communication between therapist and doctor/nutritionist, which is done with a client's consent and knowledge. If clients are motivated to change, and the problem is not severe, they can make rapid progress.

Group 4
When clients are more severely ill (e.g. weight is very low or high, extreme measures are used to control weight, or there are co-morbid symptoms), it becomes irresponsible to try and support them with therapy alone, and more intensive involvement of a GP, nutritionist and/or practice nurse becomes essential. In this case changes need to be made to the usual principle of confidentiality, and a client's approval must be sought to divulge certain information to others in the team, in order to create the best possible support.

Group 5
Therapists may get actively involved in a multi-disciplinary approach headed by a psychiatric team. It is great if the whole team operates in a solution-focused way, but in reality we come across many professionals who approach the client and their difficulty in a problem-focused manner. At best, the team can be persuaded to experiment with solution-focused interventions. At worst, there may be some suspicion about the solution-focused work being done. Thus, the therapist must tread gently. All team members will have the same goal; that is, to help the client recover. With this in mind, we can gracefully compliment others on their achievements, and be interested in what they do and how they do it. Meanwhile, a clear message is given to the client that the therapist is, and will remain, on his or her side.

Group 6
Severely ill clients do not generally present for one-to-one therapy outside a specialist unit. If weight loss is rapid and severe, the client's malnutrition prevents them being able to connect with the process. Therapy is contra-indicated but can be recommenced when nutrition has improved.

Group 7
Some clients choose not to engage in the therapeutic process. This may be because of their stage of recovery (see below) or the lack of "fit" between client and therapist. I do not think it is ethical to work with clients who do not make progress, and usually suggest they might do better with someone else, or re-commence our work when they think I can be of help.

Group 8
I have a few clients who, in spite of the severity and duration of their illness, feel that solution-focused therapy can be of help. They are trying to recover from long-term eating disorders and may elsewhere have been branded as "impossible cases". As I said before, I think clients only show resistance if the therapist has asked the wrong ques-

tion, in which case the therapist would do well to scuttle back to the drawing board. I firmly believe "No One Is Impossible", and where there is life, there is hope for improvement. As long as a client shows commitment to therapy and there are (even tiny) signs of progress, our work continues.

Clear guidelines and achievable goals must be set and it is inadvisable to work with this needy and fragile group without additional nutritional and medical support.

Clients are free to see me on their own or to bring a relative or friend. The object of the exercise is to keep the sessions flexible, and some clients choose to be accompanied for some sessions, and at other times prefer to attend on their own. Working in a solution-focused way accommodates their choices: if it works for the client we do more of it.

Stages of recovery

In thinking about clients' recovery, I have found the work of Prochasca and DiClemente (1984) very useful. They suggest that recovery weaves back and forth through five stages: pre-contemplation, contemplation, determination, action, and maintenance, as described below. Although these are generalisations, they have been in my experience invaluable for pitching the right therapeutic approach.

Every phase addresses simultaneously what clients envisage life to be like without the problem, and what they are able to eat. The object of the exercise is to break the cycle that may have started with one of the following:

– Chaotic eating (restricting/dieting/bingeing) causing a chaotic mindset, causing further chaotic eating, causing an even more chaotic mindset, etc.
– Chaotic mindset (resulting from depression/life-event) causing chaotic eating, causing a more chaotic mindset, causing an increasing chaotic eating pattern, etc.

Therapy helps to stabilise both aspects. Regular food intake will have a positive effect on the mindset, while increased equilibrium will help to establish a regular eating pattern. Alongside this, issues such as increasing self-esteem and confidence, assertiveness, positive thinking and so on, are addressed.

Pre-contemplation

Clients stuck in this phase may be reluctant to attend therapy, and doubtful that it will work. Often they have been coerced or pressured to seek help by friends or relatives, although they themselves do not accept that there is a problem.

> Sonia (14) felt press-ganged by her parents to come and see me. She said they had sent her because she did not want to eat with the rest of the family and she had been losing some weight. As far as she was concerned, there was no problem. She was happy to be thin, wasn't bothered about eating in her

bedroom, could do all the things she wanted to do, and wished they would leave her alone. Coming to see me was a positive irritation, a total waste of time.

T: I can see where you're coming from, you'd much rather be at home right now, doing computer games, so I'm wondering ... what do your mum and dad need to see happen to make them realise you no longer need to waste time here?
S: I don't know, I just wish they'd stop hassling me. Hassle, hassle, hassle. That's all I get.
T: So what do you think you could do to get them off your back?
S: I suppose they'd stop hassling me if they saw me eat something.
T: What would that be?
S: Anything really, a cereal bar or something.
T: [Surprised] A cereal bar would make a difference? How?
S: I think so. They'd see me eat and they'd be happier.
T: You would get less hassle, they would be happier ... what else would happen when you eat a cereal bar?
S: [Grunts] I'd have some energy. [Rolls eyes up to ceiling]
T: Hmm.... What could you do with that energy?
S: I'd feel happier.
T: Oh? *You'd* feel happier?
S: Hmm.
T: What difference will *that* make?

We scaled the difference that eating one cereal bar would make and predicted the improvements that would result from eating a little more. On the strength of this, we started to work on Sonia's ability to have meals with the family again, which she was able to do successfully, and after four sessions she did get mum and dad off her back.

The destructive nature of the eating disorder can be clear to the therapist and others, but clients may not want to change their eating behaviours at all. However, they *might* be prepared to use therapy to address a relationship problem, trouble at work, or some other frustration. They often make another appointment to do further work on these. Eventually, therapy may come round to focusing on the eating disorder, but on the principle that if one area improves others follow, they may find food-related problems begin to resolve "by themselves".

Paradoxically, people with severe eating disorders consider a "good day" to be a day when they have not eaten/have successfully vomited everything up/have been able to do at least six hours of intensive exercise to burn off the tiny amount they did eat. Therefore, they see no reason why they should change. At times it is possible to do some meaningful work anyway, by saying:

"OK, I appreciate that you don't think you have a problem in this area, but would you like to use the rest of this session to work on any other issues?" Sometimes clients with anorexia nervosa or bulimia nervosa are so entrenched in their wish to lose weight that they ignore the negative and dangerous implications, and cannot see that regaining even a small amount of weight would be beneficial. If they state that their goal for coming to see me is to reduce their weight even further (that is, to a dangerous level), I will explain that I am unable support them in this practice, as helping people to grow more ill would be unethical.

I invite them to make another appointment in the future if they feel that changing to a healthier lifestyle becomes a possibility and that coming back to see me would help them.

Connie (21) came to see me at her mother's insistence because of rapid weight loss. She ate very little and vomited most of that. She was obviously underweight, saying that at 5' 7" she weighed just under 50 kilos (8 stones) with clothes on. Her menstrual periods had stopped.

T: OK, Connie, so if our work together were to be successful, what would you have achieved?
C: I will have lost at least another 6 kilos.
T: So ... how would that make a difference?
C: I'd feel a lot happier and a lot more confident.
T: What would it help you do differently?
C: I'd be able to go out, enjoy myself ...
T: Hmm.... There are a few things that I don't quite understand. Can you help me out here?
C: Yeah.
T: You say your periods have stopped
C: That's obviously 'cause I'm too fat.
[Connie continued to state that if she weighed 45 kilos her periods would return because she would feel happier]
C: When I was 45 kilos I was pleased with the way I looked. And I was pleased not to have periods anyway.
T: What else was good about your life at that time?
C: I could get into all my tiny clothes.
T: What else?
C: I liked feeling my ribs and my hip bones stick out.
T: What else was good when you weighed 45 kilos?
C: Um ...

T: You're thinking hard.
C: Um ... [Long silence]
T: I'm really interested to know what we would be working towards. You know, hearing what you have to say about improving your life, I'm thinking ... are there any *other* ways we could look at to help you feel happier ... rather than through losing more weight?
C: No.
T: Sorry, I haven't got it yet, but how would your life improve when you've lost that weight?
C: I can't be arsed with all that now, I just know that I want to be 45 kilos again. Or less ... that would be even better. At the moment I'm huge and I just need to lose some weight.
T: So ... what you say is that we can't consider any other ways to get you to be happy?
C: I want you to help me lose weight. You're supposed to be the expert.
T: What I have to say is, that I will not be able to support you in this.
C: I thought you were here to help people!
T: I am here to help people get better, but ... I have a feeling that there is a difference between *your* idea of getting better and *my* idea of getting better.
C: If you say so. As far as I'm concerned, I'm perfectly OK. You're not gonna make me put on weight.
T: Alright, and I appreciate that, and if our work involved you staying the same weight as you are now? [NB once clients engage in therapy they learn to relax about weight gain, particularly if it is not made to feel the central issue of therapy]
C: I'd rather die.
T: In which case we need to discuss if it is worth you spending time here with me.
C: I don't think it is ... if you're not going to tell me how to lose more weight!

We agreed to call it a day and discussed it with her mother when she came to pick Connie up. I was very concerned about her low weight and obtained her permission to write a letter to Connie's GP in which I voiced my worries and our reasons for terminating therapy. She wanted to lose more weight and did not wish to address issues other than weight, while I felt I was not able to offer her the support she needed.

I said that in view of the seriousness of her condition she would benefit more from a structured (in-patient) re-feeding programme with intensive therapy.

Clients like Connie are stuck in the pre-contemplative stage and cannot see the benefit of change. It is important to ensure safe and ethical practice, particularly if clients are seriously ill, as Connie was. The BACP professional and ethical guidelines state that confidentiality must be broken if clients are in danger of seriously harming themselves, and severe eating distress must be seen to fall in this category.

Contemplation
Although not fully committed to counselling, contemplative clients recognise there is a problem and are willing to talk about it. There is often ambivalence about recovery: on the one hand it sounds attractive, but fear of obesity or uncertainty about living without the "support" of an eating disorder may prevent progress. Clients are encouraged to identify the discrepancies between their present situation and their preferred future. The usefulness of the eating disordered behaviour is challenged, which guides them out of the contemplation phase, as the following example shows.

> Frances (34) is a high school teacher. She suffered silently from bulimia nervosa since the age of 16, following a period of dieting. She slowly increased laxatives in order to keep her weight stable, but was beginning to suffer some serious side effects (faecal incontinence, pins and needles in hands and feet, emerging electrolyte imbalance). She felt she had reached the stage of wanting to overcome her problem. However, the thought of not taking laxatives (30 per day) filled her with terror because she was convinced she would end up putting on vast amounts of weight. This was the first time she had ever talked about her problem.

F: I know what I'm doing isn't right, but I'm scared stiff to stop because I know I'll get fat.
T: Are you satisfied with the weight you are now?
F: No, not exactly, I weigh nearly eleven stone and could do with losing some. That's why I don't think I could give up.... This weekend for instance, I'm going to a friend's wedding. There will be a buffet and I know I won't be able to control myself. What with the food and the booze.... If I didn't have the laxatives, I'd put on several pounds overnight. I'd really like to lose some weight.
T: So what you would like to happen is this: ditch the laxatives and be slimmer.
F: That's right.
T: Hang on ... there's something I don't quite understand. Are you saying that even while you take thirty laxatives a day, you're still overweight?
F: Yeah. That's right.
T: So I'm thinking that ... laxatives aren't actually such a successful method of weight loss?
F: Hmm ... I suppose they can't be.

T: There is this saying in solution-focused therapy. It goes like this: if it *doesn't* work, try something different. So, if you were not using laxatives, what other ways could you think of that might start tackling this problem?
F: [Thinks for a while] I graze a lot between meals ... I suppose I could do less of that.
T: OK ... so not grazing frees up some valuable time. How will you use that time instead?

Frances and I started challenging the usefulness of the laxatives and focused on the fact that ultimately she would like to be able to function without them. We asked questions such as, "What would be different? What else? What else?" and "What would you need to do go make a small difference?" "How likely would it be that she could make that small difference?" etc.

In the past Frances had tried unsuccessfully to cut out laxatives in one fell swoop. She agreed that she would start to reduce them slowly, while trying to graze less between meals. Increasing the calorific value of her main meals would make her feel less hungry, and so reduce the temptation to nibble. We also started focusing on her life without the problem, by addressing what she could do with her newly-found spare time.

Eating disorders tend to drive clients into isolation. It is understandable that having lived in an ivory tower for a long time, "supported" by the eating disorder and negative thought patterns, clients can be very frightened about life without their "security blanket", and there is often ambivalence about getting better. The therapist assumes a position of "not knowing", and invites the client to explain in depth the usefulness of their problem. Together, they challenge the benefits of the eating disorder and, if appropriate, new ways of thinking and being are formulated.

This ambivalent phase is a characteristic one on the road to recovery. The process may be totally baffling for the outsider, but to the person trying to recover, the eating disorder may have been a "friend" for a long time, and it would be cruel to banish it. So we might discuss how the eating disorder has had a nasty habit of sneaking up on the client, and now the client can use a similar technique: the changes are such that the eating disorder is hardly aware that it is being pushed aside. The goals have to be easily achievable to give clients the courage to push forward a little more.

Determination

This stage is marked by a client's motivation and willingness to take action in order to bring about change. Collaboratively, appropriate and meaningful goals are set. These often are based on a client's description of "exceptions"; that is, the times the problem is less severe. When clients enter therapy in this phase, progress is usually swift. This is an exciting stage, when clients begin to use their creativity to set new objectives. The scaling exercise shows a steady improvement and therapy evolves around devising more small steps to progress further along the scale.

Jodie (29) had swung from anorexia to bulimia nervosa for many years and when she first came to see me she recognised she had a severe problem. In terms of the eating disorder she felt close to 0 on the "well-being scale", yet she was at 9 on the "determination to change" scale. We discovered that the times she felt a little better were linked to when she had "something decent to eat". She responded very well to externalisation, which enabled her to make choices. She stopped mindlessly reaching for sweets and biscuits.

J: I can feel the monster sitting on my shoulder, saying, "Go on! Have that cake, have that biscuit and then go and throw up." But I know I won't feel better for that, so I just tell it to piss off, and then I have something like a sandwich instead, which makes me feel a lot better!

T: And as a result of feeling better, what can you do?

In the course of a few weeks Jodie resolved that sticking to complex carbohydrates and foods containing unsaturated fat suited her. She regulated her food intake and consequently became more even-tempered. Great improvements were made in all areas of her life. Learning to be assertive towards her "monster" made her more discerning with choices of boyfriends, and she felt she would never be used as a doormat again. After four sessions she reached the point she wanted to get to, which was being confident and able to eat a "normal" diet; that is, a wide variety of foods, including being able to enjoy the odd bar of chocolate or cake and feeling good about it.

Action

This is an extension of the previous stage. The client consistently reports changes and is meeting goals, while the therapist amplifies successes and asks appropriate solution-focused questions to find out what the client needs to do in order to maintain the progress. Most clients are getting close to the point on the scale where they initially envisaged therapy would finish.

Margaret (45) had suffered from compulsive binge eating for several years. At the start of therapy she weighed 80 kilos, and as she was only just 5' tall, this was considered overweight. She had attempted many diets but every time she finished one, she would end up putting on more weight than she had just lost. This did not do much for her self-esteem. When we first met she was feeling low, worthless, disgusted with herself and out of control. She also felt very unhealthy. We had four weekly sessions in which she learnt to replace her destructive coping strategies with constructive ways of comforting and nurturing herself. She spread the following sessions to fortnightly and monthly and after 10 sessions, having lost about 15 kilos, she felt she was sufficiently equipped to "go it alone".

In the penultimate session she bounced into my office:

M: I've had a brilliant week!
T: Ooh … tell me all about it!
M: I haven't binged at all, and I've hardly had any chocolate.… And I've not felt weak or hungry. And I've lost another three kilos! We had a barbecue and I didn't secretly eat all the left-overs.
T: Wow! Slow down … I can't keep up with you [Scribbling furiously; laughter] How did you do all that?
M: Well … after our last session I went to the supermarket to do the weekly shop. I ate a banana in the car so I wouldn't feel hungry and be tempted to get stuff that is not so good for me … came home, put it all away, and was able to put the kids' chocolate bars for their packed lunches straight into the tin. I couldn't believe it! I was so determined: these are for the kids, and not for you! Since then, I haven't touched their chocolate. It felt great!
T: That is an immense U-turn! Can you remember telling me in the first session that you'd buy a six-pack of choc bars "for the kids" and eat them before you got home, so you'd go to the corner shop to replace them?
M: Yeah … I do remember … and sometimes I'd scoff those as well, and then I'd go and get some more!
T: So on that day you put them away, you haven't touched them since. What have you been doing instead?
M: I've been making more effort with my appearance. I keep busy. And instead of slobbing around, reading the paper with several mugs of coffee and a packet of biscuits, I do something else … paint my nails, spend a lot of time in the bath just soaking … reading a book! I feel much more comfortable now I've lost weight. Having a bath is a real treat now. I enjoy life so much more … being with friends, having a coffee in town. Marcus and the kids have noticed a difference
T: What have they noticed?
M: I'm happier, more relaxed. The kids think they have a nicer mummy!
T: That sounds great. Well done. And you look radiant! Tell me … what do you think you will be able to do to circumvent any obstacles that may throw themselves at you in the future?

Margaret came up with a list of distractions to take her mind off bingeing. We looked at those in detail and celebrated her past successes. She had moved up on the scale from 4 to 6, which is where she initially hoped to finish therapy.

This stage is concerned with reiterating successes as well as exploring the future in a realistic way. There are going to be difficult times when the eating disorder lies in wait, ready to pounce on the unsuspecting client. How can this be prevented or overcome? The client is invited to prepare various coping mechanisms in advance, and if appropriate, the therapist may supplement this with practical advice.

Sometimes clients enter therapy in the action phase, like Helen, one of my research participants:

"When I decided to come and see you, I knew I didn't want to be sick anymore. But I didn't know how to do it ... and then all of a sudden I stopped. I think it started when I first rang you. I just put that barrier there. Every time I came to see you we would talk about what I had done – it was positive, it just gave me a boost, the confidence to go further."

Having suffered from anorexia and bulimia for many years, Helen moved from 3 to a steady 8-9 in five sessions that were spread over three months, and she had maintained this level at her two year follow-up.

Maintenance

In this final stage clients report consistent progress. They have stayed at a satisfactory point on the scale and can recognise behaviours that prevent relapse.

We are actively working towards ending therapy and accept that life is risky: the eating disorder will be lurking in the undergrowth, ready to pounce when stress kicks in. Possible obstacles are identified and a relapse plan is developed.

It is important to look at the client's support structure at this point. Who can they rely on when they feel they are slipping? How can they activate the skills and coping strategies they learnt before? The scales will be a useful tool to measure where they are in recovery; they have put markers along the way that will tell them when they may need to step up their vigilance.

The "open door policy" is discussed: clients are welcome to book a top-up session if they need one. I like to finish the last session with a celebration. We look back at the notes I made in the first meeting. These provide evidence of how far the client has come.

Whoops!

An awareness of these five stages certainly helps me assume the position of "not knowing" and "leading from behind"; that is, carefully monitoring how far and how fast the client is willing or able to push an issue. And however much I might wish that they move a little faster, because I can see how life would be so much better for them if only they would make certain changes, I have to sit tight and watch the picture develop at their pace. I do tell clients at the start that I can get a little carried away, and invite them to put on the breaks when that happens.

The best detective tool for catching myself being over-zealous is noticing when clients "glaze over" and begin to say, "Yes, but" a lot. This could mean:
- I have not listened to the client's goals or wishes.
- I have been too generous and have given the client an overdose of my own ideas.
- My advice/suggestions do not match the client's needs.
- I have gone too fast.
- These indulgences on my part can be easily remedied – a profuse apology usually does the trick.

Gilly (17) came to see me for support to overcome anorexia. She was also trying to reduce her alcohol intake (having been a heavy drinker since the age of twelve), and she cut her arms regularly. Her care also involved seeing her GP and a dietician. We agreed to focus on the anorexia, but one day I got waylaid and found myself "sight-seeing" around the alcohol issues. It took her about ten "Yeah, buts" before I realised that I was barking up the wrong tree. I asked if it was useful for us to sidestep into reducing the alcohol, and she politely told me that it wasn't. Thankfully she was very understanding of the fact that I'm not perfect, and accepted my apology. We were then able to do some "decent" work combating her anorexia monster. As therapy progressed and she overcame anorexia nervosa, the alcohol intake reduced, and she stopped cutting her arms without us having to wade into those waters at all.

A gradual process

Eating disorders are known to bring with them a mixture of low self-esteem, perfectionism, loss of control, depression, suspicion, superstition and feelings of being overwhelmed by the problem.

As I said before, clients often feel "stuck". Having suffered for a long time, they have a reasonable idea of what they no longer want to happen, but have no idea of what they would prefer. Thinking ahead to the time the eating disorder is not there can fill them with terror. They have long worked on the premise that they have a choice between the devil and the deep blue sea, so it's better to stick with the devil they know.

Giving little time to problem definition, solution-focused therapy quickly offers the client an opportunity to (re-)create a life without the eating disorder, or at least a life in which the problem can be much better managed.

I often invite clients to liken recovery to revamping a house. When they come to therapy their house is stuffy, full of cobwebs, dark and dingy with old-fashioned furnishings and furniture. Very few people are able to do a speedy makeover "as shown on TV" overnight. So we choose to start on one room, by removing the old and bringing in the new. Drab colours are replaced with fresh ones. A good spring clean lets the sunshine in. Uncomfortable old chairs with the springs sticking out are thrown into the skip. Replacements are bought as and when clients can afford them. And when they are ready, we can start on the next room. Just like their recovery, this is a gradual process.

Looking for evidence.
Solution-focused work is not built on pipe dreams. *Factual evidence* is extracted from the client's story and reflected back. Janice (28), a nursery school teacher with binge-eating problems, gave a wonderful example:

T: What good things have happened since we last met?
J: Oh, it's been awful. Christmas didn't do my waistline any good. I was given a huge box of chocolates, one with three layers in it … and last night I sat down, opened this box and ate two layers in one sitting.
T: *Two* layers?
J: [Hanging her head] Yeah. Disgusting.… I'm disgusted with myself for that.
T: [Amazed] *How did you do that?*
J: Yeah, you'd have thought I'd be able to control myself. I'm so ashamed …
T: No, I mean how did you stop at two layers? You could have scoffed the whole lot. In fact, when we first started working together, I remember you telling me that is exactly what you did!
J: Yeah …
T: So tell me, *how* did you decide to stop after the second layer?
J: [Thinks for a while, then perks up] Ooh… so I did! I *did* stop!
T: So … how did you do that?
J: I told myself that was enough.
T: You just *did* that!
J: [Pleased] Yeah, quite good, really, isn't it?
T: I think it's fab.… Most people say it's more difficult to stop mid-binge than not eating any chocolate at all. So this is a double whammy!

This example shows the importance of exception seeking. Concrete evidence was given to show that Janice was not as weak as she imagined, and that she was making significant progress. From feeling totally crushed, she rapidly turned herself around to owning that she had achieved something, and on the strength of this she continued making many more positive changes.

The therapist respects the function and usefulness of the problem, and assumes a position of "not knowing", with questions such as:

"So using laxatives is beneficial to you … could you help me understand how that works?"
"I'm obviously a little slow here, so humour me ·… can you explain what the

benefits are of not eating?"

"Could you just go over the comfort you get from eating such quantities of food again?"

As clients explain why they do what they do, and the benefits of their behaviour are questioned, they discover for themselves that there are big holes in their reasoning. This reconstruction process takes place at the client's pace, so it becomes less threatening to start addressing some destructive eating-disordered behaviours. Furthermore, the "letting go" process is carefully balanced with the process of taking on new, positive attitudes and coping mechanisms. Thus, clients do not feel that letting go of the eating disorder is like being pushed over a cliff.

In solution-focused therapy, attention is given to detail. Global expressions such as "I just want to be normal" are followed up with:

"Just so I can understand you better, could you explain what exactly does 'being normal' mean for you? What will you be doing differently? What else? What else?"

A new way of being begins to unfold. A life of limitation, seclusion, fear, suspicion, fatigue and food-focusing transforms into a life of opportunity, inclusion, confidence, trust, energy and interest in things other than food.

Externalisation

In June 1999 I attended a workshop given by the Australian narrative therapist Michael White, and I learnt about the benefits of "externalisation" (White & Epson, 1990). I started to incorporate this into my work. Both solution-focused therapy and narrative therapy originate in post-modern philosophy, which is why I think that, although externalisation is not strictly speaking a solution-focused intervention, it can quite comfortably be used alongside this model.

I would like to explain how the narrative concept can be used to help people overcome an eating disorder.

Many of my clients state that they *are* the problem: "I *am* an anorexic/a bulimic/a compulsive binge eater." This makes me feel so sorry for them. Fancy having to go through life with a millstone like that around your neck!

They often describe the eating disorder as "a tight feeling within my chest," and I invite them to gently remove it and to put it on their shoulder instead. In this way they have separated themselves from the problem. And rather than spending valuable time trying to change the client, it gives us the opportunity to form an alliance against the eating disorder, the "monster" that has invaded their life. Clients are invited to get others to join the fight. This results in dramatic changes in relationships as a mother of a ten-year-old explained:

"Before we learnt about the 'monster', it felt that we were battling against Poppy … so much stress, hurt, anger. But now, when she runs into difficulties like not wanting to eat, or being rude, we can say, 'Do I see Slimy Toad creeping up on your shoulder? Shall we try and push him off together? Let's put him outside the kitchen door so you can get on with your meal!' And we have a giggle about Slimy Toad trying to get at her but not being able to! We have a common enemy. Somehow it has brought us closer together. The other benefit is that once we identified the monster that attached itself to her, we can see our lovely child again. And we concentrate on the times that we see more of her, and less of her monster. It's become quite a game lately … we can even laugh about it now!"

Some clients give their monster a name or describe what it looks like, others have found it helpful to draw it. We imagine that it behaves like a jealous lover. It wants the client all to itself, and has devious ways of going about its job. Depending on the type of eating disorder, it could whisper into the client's ear something like this:

The anorexic monster: "Don't eat, and you will feel better!"
The bulimic monster: "Eat that packet of biscuits! You'll enjoy it and you can always chuck it up/take laxatives/exercise it off afterwards."
The compulsive binge-eating monster: "Why don't you just have that loaf of bread and butter, a bucket of ice cream and those twelve bars of chocolate? You know it will soothe you!"
The yo-yo diet monster: "Just eat those goodies, and we'll start another diet tomorrow!"
The athletica nervosa monster: "You must exercise today, or you'll get flabby!"
The restrictive-eating/difficulty-in-swallowing monster: "If you eat that you will die."
The orthorexia monster: "You just stick to your carrots, you are the wise one, the virtuous one … leave them to silt up their arteries with fat and sugar!"
The chew-spit monster: "Enjoy the taste, the flavour, the feel of it…. But don't swallow at any price, or you'll put on a vast amount of weight!"

In therapy, clients learn to question such lies, threats and promises, and these techniques are used between sessions. The conversation below illustrates how a client successfully challenges an anorexia monster.

C: I fancy an apple.
M: If you eat that apple, you will lose control and you won't be able to stop eating! You will eat the whole fruit basket. You'll end up getting fat. I tell you what: don't eat *anything* … then you'll feel in control, and you *know* you like feeling in control.
C: One apple is not going to make me fat. I know I don't have to eat all that

fruit because I managed to just have one apple yesterday ... and what's more, eating a little something actually made me feel better.

The client decides to eat the apple. In the game of recovery the score is Client:1 – Monster: 0.

C: I think I might go out with my friends this evening.
M: Oh no, don't go out with them! They don't love you ... it's much better if you stay here at home, with me, nice and safe. Stay here with me, just you and I together. I will make sure that no one can hurt you, no one can touch you.
C What evidence do you have that they don't love me? Why would they keep ringing me and asking me out if they didn't like me?
M: They are only pretending, they don't really mean it....
C: Give me evidence.
M: They don't really care about you at all. In fact, no one cares about you, so you're much better off here, with me.
C If I stay at home I'll be alone and miserable.
M: Ah, but just think of the implications of going out ... think of the drink and the food they will want to force on you. Think of the calories! If you go out you will totally lose control and you will be as big as a house in the morning.
C: Last time I went out I managed OK with a salad and some mineral water. They did not force anything on me, *and* I did not put on any weight.
M: But if you stay here with me, you will feel great ... you will feel totally in control
C: So how will that benefit me?
M: You *know* you like that feeling of being totally in control.
C: You are telling me a lie! If I stay here, *you* will be in control and I will be miserable! I'd rather take a risk and go out. There is more chance that I will have a good evening when I'm with my friends. I may feel in control when I don't eat, but what will happen as a result? Starving makes me weak and hungry, lonely and miserable. That does not feel good at all, so I'm off and you can stay here!

The client goes out for the evening and the score is Client: 2 – Monster: 0.
Looking for exceptions and externalising work well in tandem. For example, Bill has a chew-spit habit. He is convinced that if he swallows *anything* he will put on weight.

T: I wonder if you could clarify something for me.... You say you can't swallow *anything*.

B: Yeah. I just can't ... because if I do, I'll get fat.
T: Your monster is telling you that you'll end up as big as a "Martello" tower if you swallow *anything*?
B: Yeah! [Laughter]
T: But could you just clarify something for me ... because if you don't eat *anything*, how come you had the energy to get here today?

This enabled Bill to look at the few things he was able to swallow, which was evidence that swallowing food was not synonymous with piling on weight. This enabled him to extend his food repertoire. This increased his energy, lifted his mood and made him more confident socially.

Initially it can be difficult to differentiate between "monster-talk" and "client talk". Monsters can be very sneaky, pretending really to care for the well-being of the client, as this example shows:

The client is trying to stabilise her intake, has been able to have a reasonable meal, and then starts thinking, "Go on! Eat some more, you haven't had enough!" It pays at this point to take time out to evaluate what she has eaten (e.g. a sandwich, piece of fruit and yoghurt for lunch). As this is genuinely sufficient, she can identify that the monster is trying to persuade her to have more.

C: I do not need any more, I have eaten enough. I am able to stop now.
M: Eat some more, because if you stop now, you have not had enough (for me to persuade you to throw up/exercise/abuse laxatives/feel guilty and out of control).

Externalising the eating disorder gives clients the opportunity to be angry with the monster rather than with themselves. It paves the way for self-nurturing and increasing self-esteem. It also opens up a new world of choices. One of my clients discovered it in this way:

"Working in this way has made me realise something: recovery is all about choices and trust. I use these words like a mantra during the day: 'I have choices, I have choices.' For so long the eating disorder has made choices for me, and I have just followed meekly behind. And when I make a choice (for instance: 'I will eat a sandwich instead of not eating at all') I need to trust myself at having made the right one, and trust my body that it's not going to fail me by blowing up like a balloon as a result."

Ben (45), a care assistant, had suffered from bulimia nervosa since his mid-twenties. Several times a week he would drink an entire bucket of soapy water after his meal to help him vomit everything up. His story was horrifying. He had been badly abused by his boorish father who was widowed when Ben was twelve. Being the eldest he was expected to leave school and look after his father and five siblings. When we evaluated our work he said:

"Once I got the hang of 'monster talk' I could separate myself from the past. I stopped wallowing in how bad things were … I never realised I had a choice in the matter before. I just knew I had to be clean and I had to do this [drink soapy water and be sick]. I needed to be good, and clean … I suppose I tried to wash the old man out. But you showed me that I wasn't being very effective. And that I had a choice! I don't need to let the memory of my dad and his nastiness cast a shadow on my future. It's much better living my life doing justice to my mum's memory, be healthy… look forward…. She certainly wouldn't want me to suffer like I have."

Having been under the thumb of the eating disorder has made clients forget how to be discerning, but once they start externalising they can say:

"Well, Monster, this may be what you want me to do, and making me do that may well suit you! But I don't want to go along with this any longer, so instead I will do X …Y… Z.…"

This is a very powerful experience. Starting with small choices that bring about small changes, the client soon finds the courage to make bigger choices, which results in a steady move up the scale. Separating the monster from the client also gives the therapist the opportunity to highlight the good side of the client's character, which most people in eating distress fail to see themselves. Clients gradually choose to accept that they are valued and precious members of society.

Clients generally agree that they would not wish the eating disorder on their worst enemy, so it stands to reason that no one, not even they, deserve to be imprisoned by it. Their increased ability to do justice to themselves and be assertive towards the monster begins to affect other areas in their lives as well. It is exciting to see withdrawn clients blossom. As they overcome the restricting powers of their monster, they also begin to stand up to those who kept them in their subservient role.

Externalising enables clients to stop beating themselves up, which leaves time and space for self-nurturing and enjoying life. For some, making moves in recovery involves "forgiving themselves for what they have done." Liz expressed the following:

"If you don't manage to detach the eating disorder, you just think: '*I've* got myself here, now *I've* got to suffer the consequences. I've made my own life a misery, and that of everyone around me. All I deserve is a slow, painful death.' But when you suggested, 'Let's just think of this as something external, so we can n fight against it together,' recovery then became almost like a game … it made things so much more light-hearted! And less overwhelming. If, inside, you still think, 'Oh well, you don't deserve anything good to happen to you, because you did this to yourself,' you're *never* going to get better, because you'll *never* be able to forgive yourself for what you've done

'Monster-bashing Methods'

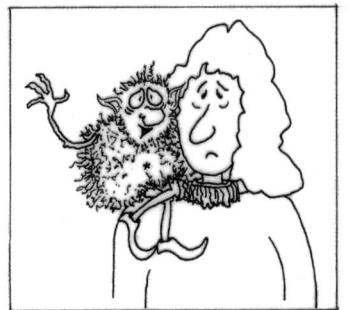

'Help! There's a monster on my shoulder...'

Give him a direct line (in one ear - out the other)

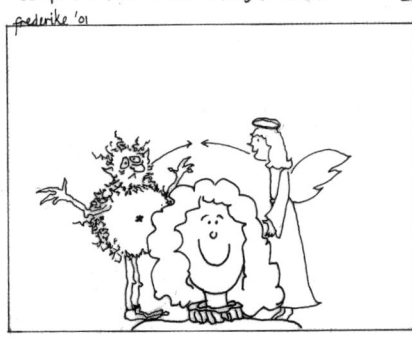

Set your guardian-angel on him

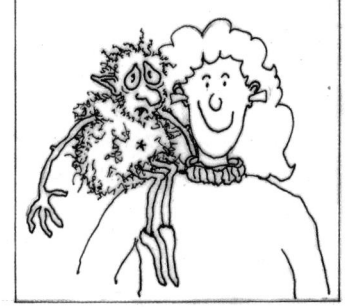

Use earplugs

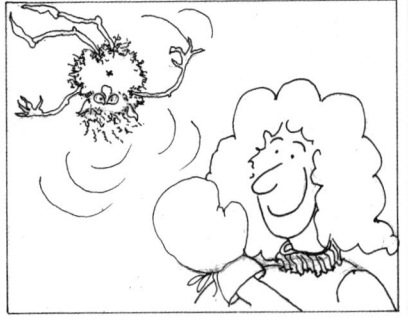

Box him off

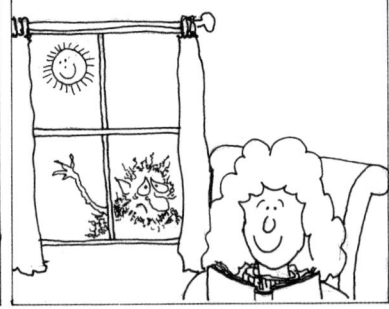

Create a 'monster-free zone'

Turning "failures" into "successes"

A refreshing way of approaching the "downs" of recovery is not to dwell on the times when the client slipped. We are not interested in the details of how and why, it is sufficient to know that it happened. What we are interested in is this: how do clients turn themselves around? (Berg, 1993)

C: I went right down to a 2 over the weekend. I binged and vomited several times. I wanted to go out wearing my little miniskirt but I decided I looked fat and frumpy in it, and, well ... that was it. I just had to punish myself!
T: So you slipped down to a 2 ... and how long did you stay there?
C: Several days.
T: That must have been horrible. How come you didn't slip any further?
or:
T: But then, I notice, you moved up the scale. How did you do that?
or:
T: What gave you the strength to turn yourself around? (What else? What else?)

In this way we acknowledge how bad it has been for the client, but firmly discredit the power of the "failures" and celebrate the successes instead. We closely follow the client's progress up the scale, monitoring what they are doing that works. In effect, we are turning failures into successes (Berg).

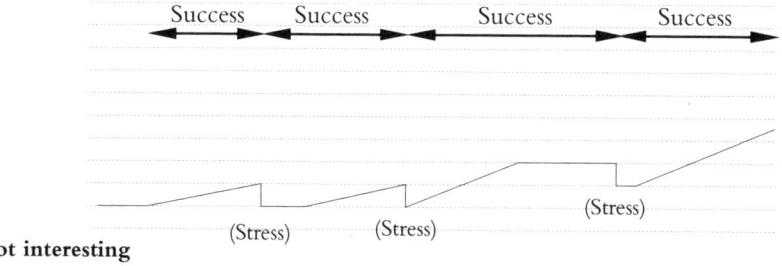

From rigid routines to flexibility

Eating disorders of the restricting kind have a knack of seducing people into the "safety" of rigid routines. Meal times are set and food planning is done with meticulous precision, and if for any reason the strict boundaries come under threat, it can cause major emotional upset. We address the false sense of security that is offered by this rigidity and begin to move towards being flexible and spontaneous around food. This may mean temporarily taking on board other, less destructive "routines".

A dietician may suggest a meal plan which initially may give the client a great sense of security, knowing that at certain times each day he or she is expected to eat a certain food. I am often told that this helps to "allow" the client to eat something, which over-rides the usual restrictions. The meal plan is regularly adapted to keep in step with the pace of recovery.

Some people temporarily cut out "trigger" foods or drinks, such as chocolate, wheat, fat-saturated foods, coffee, tea or alcohol. This is best done under supervision as it can lead to malnutrition.

The key words here are "temporary" and "means to an end". We are using temporary alternatives to work towards increased flexibility. Healthy routines serve to support us. Eating breakfast, lunch and dinner at roughly the same time each day not only gives us regular fuel, it also provides a framework around which we may plan our activities. The client's ultimate goal is to be relaxed around food and enjoy a varied diet. When that happens, clients have taken on board the knowledge that "a little of what you fancy does you good."

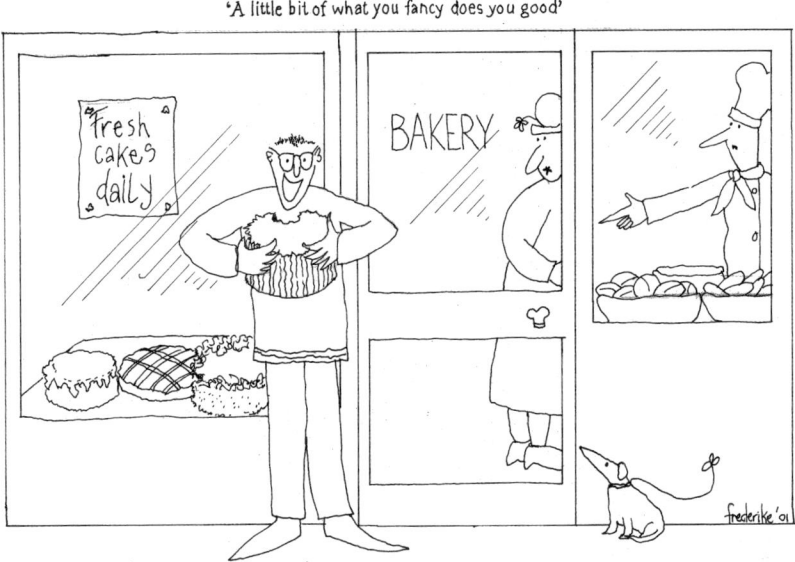

'A little bit of what you fancy does you good'

"Well, she *did* say one cake a day would be ok...."

From mindless to mindful.

I have found that solution-focused therapy is useful in helping clients exchange mindless, out-of-control and destructive feelings for mindful and purposeful ones that build self-control, assertiveness and self-esteem.

Clients tell me that eating disorders are expert at giving them an "out-of-body experience": their body appears engrossed in a full-blown binge, while their mind is hovering in the corner, looking on aghast but unable to stop it. At the other end of the spectrum, a starving client may truly wish to eat something but the eating disorder simply prevents it. These situations are often described as, "It comes over me like a wave," or "There is nothing I can do to stop/change it." In other words, the *eating disorder* is perceived to be in control. The therapist uses solution-focused questions to look for times that the *client* has shown signs of control, and this evidence is built upon.

HALT

A friend who helps people overcome alcohol dependency introduced me to an intervention called the "HALT" method, which is a useful tool to help clients get back in the driving seat. The following example illustrates the sequence of events for someone with binge eating problems. When clients feel a binge coming on, they stall it by saying "HALT!" **H** stands for hungry, **A** for angry, **L** for lonely and **T** for tired. They identify what the binge would be in aid of, and choose to use a different coping strategy instead:

H Am I *Hungry?*
   If yes:
   What kind of food would do my body justice? (A bar of chocolate may seem attractive, but clients have recognised that the benefit is short-lived)
   Mindful action:
   Choose a nurturing food to eat. Eat mindfully, and remove yourself from temptation.

A Am I *Angry?* (aka *frustrated*)
   If yes:
   Instead of a binge, what would be a useful way to deal with this anger?
   Mindful action:
   Find a different way of venting it, e.g. assertively address the problem/person causing the aggravation, blow off steam by taking a healthy walk, talking to someone about it, showing a "water off a duck's back" attitude, etc.

L Am I *Lonely?* (aka *bored*)
   If yes:
   How can I feel more included?
   Mindful action:
   Find someone to talk to; see or telephone a friend, occupy your mind with things other than food: watch a film, read a book, clean out a cupboard, pursue a hobby, etc.

T Am I *Tired?*
   If yes:
   How can I feel more energetic? (This is the trickiest one, for people

often eat sweets to give them energy and then fall into the binge-trap.)
Mindful action:
Establish that the tiredness is not caused by hunger. Think, "When was the last time I ate something decent?" Instead of eating for energy, relieve tiredness by putting your feet up, taking forty winks, going to bed early, getting some fresh air, working on the premise that "a change is as good as a rest," and do something totally different that will give you a sense of satisfaction/achievement.

The questions can be adapted to suit the various forms of eating disorders. For someone recovering from anorexia nervosa, it could be:

Am I *Hungry?*
If yes:
   What can I do that would do my body justice?
Mindful action:
Eat food that you consider to be good for your body and mind.

I feel fat

This is the most common expression heard from people with restricting eating habits and athletica nervosa. I have learnt to accept what they say; although it is plain to see that they do not *look* fat, they certainly do *feel* fat. It is pointless to say, "But of course you are not fat, look, you are wearing a size 6!" This is in fact the quickest way to make the client feel misunderstood. I have found it useful to approach the problem from another angle: I explain that it is natural to feel bloated after a (small) meal if because of having eaten little/vomited a lot/abused laxatives for a while. The stomach has shrunk and it will need to be gently eased back into shape. Small, nourishing meals will assist the process, particularly if the *client* decides what can be eaten.

My clients have also taught me that "I feel fat" is eating-disordered language for "I experience tension/stress". By focusing on food/body shape, this tension can be successfully repressed. The HALT method can be used to address these stressful issues, which then helps the client reach for constructive ways to deal with the problem.

How do I eat?

The HALT intervention also buys the client valuable time to consider the difference between mindless and mindful eating. The table below shows how my clients identify the difference between the mindless eating in a life beset by an eating disorder, and the benefits experienced from eating mindfully.

Mindless eating	Mindful eating
Eating "on the hoof" or standing up	Eating whilst sitting down, preferably at a table
Grabbing and stabbing at anything	Choosing what to have
Using hands	Using cutlery

Tired tastebuds	Taste-buds alive
Stuffing the food down	Chewing carefully
Eating alone or in front of TV	Eating alone but away from distractions, or eating with others
Secrecy about what and how much is consumed	Openness and honesty
Treats lead to binges	Treats are enjoyed
Eating quickly	Eating slowly
Not knowing how much has been consumed	Putting food on a plate, and so being aware of the portion
Food is high in refined sugar and saturated fat	Food is high in complex carbohydrates and contains unsaturated fat
Food consumed is considered unhealthy	Food consumed is considered healthy
Sense of letting oneself down (self-abuse)	Sense of doing oneself justice
No sense of enjoyment	Enjoying and savouring what is eaten
Feeling the food is not enough	Sense of contentment
Sense of loss of control	Feeling in control
Eating is followed by feeling bloated and uncomfortable	Eating is followed by feeling satisfied and comfortable
Eating is followed by feelings of self-loathing	Eating has produced "feel-good factor"
Measures taken to compensate (starving, vomiting, laxative abuse, exercising)	Relax, as compensation not required.
Not good	Good

Turning negatives into positives

When clients are low on the scale, their circumstances often resemble pure devastation. Stuck in negative thought patterns with little or no self-esteem, their metabolism is disrupted and they feel a physical wreck living in isolation and shame with a sense of total loss of control. Everything is black.

Driven by the solution-focused assumptions that "nothing is constant, change is ongoing, and there are always times that the problem is slightly less bad," (de Shazer) the therapist, like a forensic scientist, doggedly hunts for signs of competence and exceptions in the client's ravaged life. These are reflected back to the client to help in climbing out of a slough of despondency.

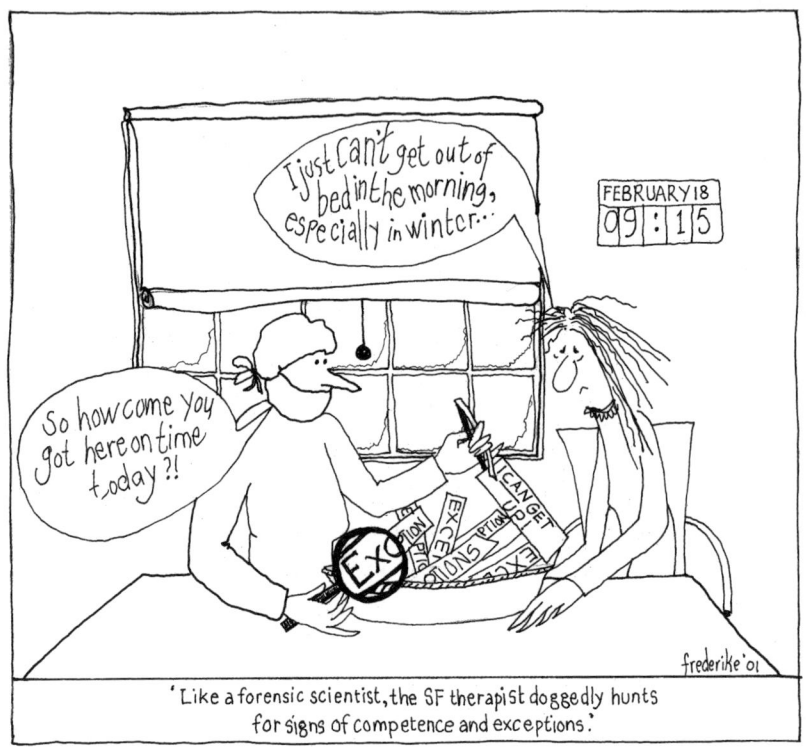

'Like a forensic scientist, the SF therapist doggedly hunts for signs of competence and exceptions.'

Eating disorders cover clients in a thick black cloak, preventing them seeing any glimmer of hope. But little by little they learn to peel it off to reveal their preferred future, the way they wish to lead their life once the monster has been banished. The case studies in the next chapter show a wealth of creativity and courage as my clients turn hopeless situations into hopeful ones.

4.

CASE STUDIES

The majority of my clients are female, aged between eighteen and forty-five, and they mainly suffer from bulimia nervosa. For the purpose of this book, and to give a broader insight into the journey of recovery, I have chosen a cross-section of my client group. Some accounts are transcripts of sessions, while others rely on written notes. To give a clear insight into the sequence of events, I have given the full transcript of Vic's therapy in Case Study 1, but the other stories are abbreviated. I start the first session by recording personal details such as name, address, date of birth and any medication clients may be taking. I explain that, if I am concerned about the health of my clients, I shall ask their permission to liaise with other health professionals and make a note of the GP or any other medical/therapeutic support. Clients are given a brief explanation of solution-focused therapy so they understand what they are letting themselves in for. An agreement on confidentiality is made and there is time for them to ask questions. I do not usually have prior knowledge or details of their illness or circumstances, nor do I request referral letters.

When I wrote up these case studies, I was struck by the unpredictability and immediacy of therapy. In solution-focused work it is agreed that clients present a problem and therapists choose to look in the opposite direction; that is, towards the preferred future. But as we do so, what makes us decide to pick up on *this* particular word or *that* particular expression? Why do we choose to explore *these* aspects in preference to *those*?

Specific needs vary from client to client and from moment to moment. What I focus on within a session may differ vastly from what others would do, and what is of therapeutic interest to one person may be abhorrent to, or simply bore the pants off, the next. I may get it wrong, and be found to be barking up the wrong tree (in which case clients hopefully put me right), or we notice that they are not making the desired progress. At worst, they may decide not to come back.

But when my clients indicate that I get it right, then I will do more of it, and continue to do so until it is no longer useful. The ultimate goal all therapists strive towards is to work with clients who make progress and are satisfied with the outcome of therapy, and I think solution-focused therapy helps us to celebrate the individuality of people. So with all this in mind I invite you to have a peep at the work that I do. Your constructive criticism and questions will be warmly received.

Case study 1: "Choc-Fix"
Victor (28)
Diagnosis: bulimia nervosa
Referral route: GP
Setting: GP surgery
Number of sessions: 9
Medication: Fluoxetine (Prozac), 40mg
Stated weight at start of therapy: 120kg.
Stated weight at end of therapy: 96 kg
Scale at start: 2. Lowest point ever: 0. Scale at finish: 7
Follow-up 2 months: 8. Follow-up 4 months: 8.5

Session 1

Pre-session change
T; So, Victor, let's make a start.
V: You can call me Vic.
T: Vic. OK, did you have to wait long for this appointment?
V: Hmm, about three weeks.
T: OK ... and in those three weeks, have you noticed any positive changes?
C: Uh ... how do you mean?
T: Well, have you thought, "Oh well, that wasn't too bad today," or, "I coped a little better with this"?
V: I see. Hmm. [Spends some time in thought] Uh ... I guess I've been looking forward to coming here ... sounds silly.... But I have. I feel that at last there is someone who is going to help me. The GP told me that you specialise in this sort of thing.
T: So a sense of starting to sort things out ...
V: Yeah. That's it.
T: And how has that been helpful?
V: I think it has been helpful. It has made me start to think.
T: Think about?
V: Think about how fed up I am about being like this. The vomiting, bingeing

...
T: I see. And has this thinking that you did before coming here resulted in you *doing* something differently?
V: Not really ... maybe. Maybe it has stopped me vomiting once or twice. Not much really.
T: But just thinking about coming here has encouraged you to vomit less in these three weeks leading up to your appointment?
V: Hmm.
T: Is that a positive change?
V: I hadn't thought of it like that.

Problem-free talk
T: OK, Vic, just so I can get to know you a little, could you describe yourself to me, things that you do, interests, hobbies, family, job.... Things that make you tick.
V: Well, I've had this problem for three years ...
T: A long time eh? But can we leave the problem to one side for a bit, 'cause I want to get to know *you* first, and we'll talk about what brought you here shortly.
V: OK ... so, what makes me tick. Well I am 28.... I have two jobs. An office job in the day, and at night I am a bouncer at a nightclub in town, three or four nights a week.
T: Do you enjoy your work?
V: I used to, but now I find it difficult, because I keep on going to the vending machine, stuffing my face with chocolate. Pressures at work are rising as well.... But yeah, I like my evening job. Meeting people ... my workmates are nice there. Keeps me occupied.
T: What are your interests? Hobbies?
V: Don't have many really. I like watching films, and I like reading.
T: Anything in particular?
V: Science fiction mainly ... detectives. I used to like swimming until I put on all this weight.
T: Swimming ... what else?
V: I like cars, but since I split with my girlfriend I've had to trade down, to get some money to furnish my flat.
T: Uh-huh. What about relatives ... friends?
V: My mum lives nearby, I see her regularly. We get on fine. My dad died when I was 19, and I have a younger sister. She is married and lives in Australia. I have a few good mates, we go to the pub together and I play darts.
T: Darts ... sounds good! Are you in a team?

V: I used to be, and I was good at it. But now I have to work a lot of evenings so I just have a go when I get the chance.
T: Anything else you enjoy that you are good at?
V: Hmm, I like DIY. You know, pottering around the flat, fixing things.

Problem definition

T: OK, thanks for that, this gives me a bit of a picture of you. Can you tell me about why you have come here today?
V: Well, the doctor suggested it because I'm bulimic.
T: I see.
V: I've been a bulimic for the past three years. It started when my girlfriend and I were having problems. She was always henpecking me, going *on,* and *on* … and then I'd binge and binge. Then I started to put on weight and she was even more disgusted with me. After I left her I started vomiting and exercising and I lost all the weight I had put on, and more. And I started eating less. But over the past year or so I'm getting more bulimic, I seem to have "lost it" and I just want to eat and eat and I have put on several stone. I vomit several times a day.
T: Several times?
V: Yeah, sometimes six, seven, eight times or more.
T: So you have been suffering from bulimia for a while and you feel it's getting worse?
V: Yeah. I have no control anymore.
T: Yet you still manage to keep up two jobs?
V: It's getting more difficult. Now I vomit several times at the office, it's doing my head in.
T: Doing your head in?
V: Yeah, the pressure of trying to bring the food up. It gives me headaches. All I think about is food, food, food. Can't concentrate on anything else! If I'm not careful they'll give me the sack.
T: Is there anyone you talk to about this? You know, people who help you, support you?
V: The first time I ever talked about it was with the doctor the other week. I don't want *anyone* to know about it. Even my mum doesn't know what's going on.
T: OK, I see. And if therapy was to turn out useful for you, what would we achieve?
V: I want to understand *why* I am a bulimic. I want to be normal. I want to stop bingeing and vomiting all the time …
T: So, let me I get it right…. You want to get rid of bulimia nervosa?

V: Yeah. That's it.

Miracle Question

T: Now, I'd like to understand what "normal" means to you, and I have a bit of an unusual question.... So you'll have to humour me.
V: That's OK. Fire away.
T: OK then, it goes like this. It is a normal evening, you do what you normally do. Then you go to bed, and while you are asleep a miracle happens, and the problem you brought here has been resolved! Now, you wake up the next morning, not knowing that the miracle has happened, 'cause you were fast asleep. What I would like to know is, what will be the *first* thing you notice as you wake, that tells you things are different?
V: So I'm no longer bulimic?
T: It's your miracle! So if you choose no longer to suffer from bulimia....
V: Well ... I'd feel normal!
T: What does normal look like?
V: Well, I'm not worrying about going to work. I'm not worrying about when I can get my hands on chocolate.
T: OK, so what are you thinking about instead?
V: I might even be looking forward to getting up.
T: What happens next?
V: I get up and shower.
T: What's different about that on this Miracle Day?
V: I'm not disgusted with myself.
T: So you're not disgusted but ...
V: A real miracle, is it?
T: Yep.
V: Well, if it is a real miracle, then I will have lost some weight and I feel pleased with myself.
T: What else happens?
V: I get dressed and go to work.
T: Without breakfast?
V: I never have breakfast.
T: And on the Miracle Day?
V: Well, another miracle would be that I'm up early enough to have some! [Laughter]
T: What do you choose?
V: Cereal, I think. And juice and coffee. Read the paper.
T: Sounds nice.
V: It does...

T: And next?
V: I go to work. Car starts straight away and I don't stop off at the garage for chocolate. And I've managed to pack up a lunch at home. So I know what I'm gonna have for lunch.
T: Wow! Loads of things are happening. What's next?
V: I get to work and get going.
T: Who will be the first to notice that this miracle has happened?
V: The tea lady, because I don't raid her trolley at eleven o'clock. [Laughter]
T: Do your colleagues notice anything different?
V: Yeah, they notice I'm not so grumpy.
T: So what do they notice instead?
V: I'm less jumpy because I don't have to raid the chocolate machine, or borrow money off them. And they will notice that I've lost weight. [Laughter]
T: What else?
V: Less grumpy.
T: *Less* grumpy and *more* ... what?
V: Talkative, uh, joking....
T: What do you do at lunch?
V: I eat my "pack-up" and I don't have to go to the loo to sick it up.
T: What do you do instead?
V: I don't sit on my own, stuffing my gob.
T: So what *do* you do?
V: Sit with the lads, have a chat, do a computer game.
T: What's that like?
V: It's fun, we're having a laugh and a joke.
T: Sounds like you're having a good time ... How does the rest of the day develop?
V: Much the same really. Go home, cook a meal, not too much. Eat it, don't vomit, get changed, go to the nightclub for evening job.
T: Will anyone there notice that a miracle has happened?
V: I'm more chatty, more cheerful, thinner! And I have more patience with the customers. I don't have to keep fretting, wanting to eat something but not being able to, 'cause I can't be sneaking off to be sick.
T: A huge change then, on this Miracle Day!
V: You're telling me!

Scaling

T: OK, Vic, what we can do now, is make a scale. [Draws horizontal line on paper, 0 on left, 10 on right; shows client] 0 represents the pits, the worst things could ever be or even *have* been. 10 is your Miracle Day. Where would

you say you are now?
V: At this moment? I would say at 2.
T: OK, have you been lower than a 2?
V: Definitely. I've been at 0.
T: That sounds bad. When was that?
V: When I was still with my girlfriend. She would belittle me and make me feel like shit. And I was comfort eating and piling on the weight. I cried constantly … a real mess. I thought things couldn't get much worse.
T: That sounds bad. So how have you managed to get from 0 to 2?
V: Leaving her helped a lot. But, well, I have been a lot higher actually, when I was at my thinnest, after we split. Must have been, well … a 10.
T: What was going on to get you at 10?
V: I was thin and confident.
T: So what were you doing to be thin?
V: Eating nothing, exercising, swimming every day …
T: A busy schedule.
V: Yeah, I wore myself out!
T: I just wanted to check something I don't quite understand … bit dim today. [Laughter] But, uh, eating nothing helped you to get thin?
V: That's right, yeah.
T: But … I'm a bit puzzled here 'cause that doesn't sound like much fun to me, bearing in mind that most socialising happens around food and drink. How did that work for you?
V: Hmm? Don't know what you mean.
T: What did you do when you were out and about, being thin and confident … when you were out with your mates?
V: I went out, had a good time …
T: A good time, yet eating *nothing*? And what about the calories in the drinks? How did you cope with all that?
V: Yeah, see what you mean. Actually, that part wasn't much fun. [Thinks a while] I started not being able to go out because there always was food around, or drink … calories. Couldn't have any of that, I had to avoid that, so I was getting a bit lonely.
T: So being thin felt good, but the way you went about it … a bit dubious?
V: Yeah … and then I seemed to lose control. Comfort eating and all that, I piled on the weight again. Look at me now, I'm disgusted with myself. I feel ashamed of myself. My trousers are tight … I couldn't be seen dead in swimming trunks. I have stretch marks on my belly and on my legs … never had those before. They itch like hell. I'm disgusting. I'm fed up. I feel useless. I'm right where I started. [Tears welling up] I think I must be going mad!

T: [Quiet for a while] A few things to pick up on here. Firstly, when your body has been put through a period of intensive exercise and starvation, it cries out for nutrition and this can be too much. So the response may be bingeing, or bulimia nervosa. This is really quite common.
V: You mean others have the same problem?
T: Loads of people are in the same boat, yes.
V: That's a relief. I thought I must be going bonkers … thought I'd end up in a nuthouse. I couldn't tell anyone what was going on, 'cause they'd lock me away if they knew. I've been feeling that bad.
T: Hmm! It *can* feel pretty bad. But what I'm interested in is that you've managed not to go as deep as you were before. Right down to a 0.
V: No, not as bad as that. I don't blubber all the time. A bit tearful maybe but no, not as bad.
T: How have you prevented getting as low as that again?
V: My nightclub job helps. I enjoy that.
T: So meeting with people in the evening helps? And the routine, having something to do?
V: Hmm. You see, it's easy there 'cause I just can't binge and vomit.
T: That sounds as if this is an achievement that shouldn't count?
V: Well, I just *can't* do it there, can I?
T: I'm not sure how this works for you. From where I stand I'd say you *choose to put yourself* in a safe environment where you can't binge and vomit. Correct me if I'm wrong, but this must be kind of a good sign?
V: Put it like that, I suppose I'm getting *something* right.
T: Hmm. Can we just nip back to our scale.… Where would you put yourself *now?*
V: So, now, I had gone right down, to 1. But talking like this, that brings me to 2. 'Cause I can see I am *doing* something!
T: Wow, so all these recent difficulties, yet you managed to hang in there at 1?
V: Hmm.
T: And even just in this session, you have gone up a point?
V: Yeah, it's useful. It gives me hope that I can get better.
T: OK. So say the work that we do has been successful and at some point you come in and say, "Thanks very much, Frederike, I no longer need to come here." How high on the scale do you think you'll be?
V: Quite high. At least a 7.
T: So what will be happening at a 7? How will we know that we've got there?
V: I won't be bingeing anymore and I will be vomiting less, maybe once a week. I will be more confident. I will have lost some weight – quite a lot actually. My boss will be happy 'cause I'll be doing better work … yeah. I'll have more

energy all round. I'll be doing something like swimming or cycling … maybe even have myself a new girlfriend?

T: OK, Vic, that's a good list to be getting on with. Now we know what we are working towards.

Compliments

T: Looking at what we have discussed today, although generally speaking you say your life is in a mess, you do find "safe places" where you can't binge-vomit. I am really impressed at your determination to sort this out. It has been a difficult and depressing time for you, yet you have been able to crawl up the scale from 0 to 2! Another thing was that you had the strength to escape from your girlfriend [Vic smiles], and that makes me think that you have the skills to get out of unwanted situations. Breaking up with your girlfriend is like breaking up with your eating disorder?

V: Hmm!

T: What I picked up on, as well, was that your Miracle Day and your scale seem very realistic. You don't seem to be asking for the moon … you are content with getting to get to a 7. Do you feel it is achievable? You know, getting to 7?

V: In time, I think so, yes.

T: OK. Now, what we need to look at is *how* are we going to get to 7?

V: Exactly. I haven't a clue….

T: OK, can I suggest we try it in very small steps? Set goals that are achievable without too much trouble?

V: OK.

Homework task

T: So between now and our next appointment, what do you think you could change?

V: I'm gonna try not to binge at all. And I will try not to vomit.

T: [Jokingly] Hang on, hang on, *panic!* [Laughter] That's a *huge* leap! From 2 to 7 in one fell swoop, eh? Shall we try and keep it small this week?

V: Uh, I dunno.

T: OK, looking at your Miracle Day…. Is there anything that strikes you that you could try and incorporate, maybe for one day or one *part of a day,* and see how it goes?

V: Well, I think I could try. One day. Hmm … I think I could try and get up early enough to have some breakfast and not stop at the petrol station for chocolate.

T: OK. So on this one occasion you want to achieve three things: getting up

earlier, having breakfast, then not buying chocolate on the way. So, if we scaled this and said 0 is a snowball in hell's chance and that at 10 you will definitely get up early one day this week, where would you pitch the chance of you doing this?
V: Quite high.
T: Where?
V: Just one day, you say?
T: Yes.
V: I'd say ... 9 or 10.
T: OK, so we can say it is very likely that between now and next session you will have got up, had breakfast, and hit the workplace without pockets bulging with chocolate, once.
V: Yes.
T: Great. What I would like you to do is to monitor very carefully what difference this makes to *that* day, or to *that* morning.
V: I can do that.
T: Great. Is there anything you wanted to address before we finish?
V: No, I think we've covered a lot.
T: Right, it was good to meet you today Vic, good luck, and see you next week.

Evaluation of session 1
In this session I carefully assessed the severity of Vic's condition. He was suffering badly from bulimia nervosa (vomiting 8 times per day gives rise for concern), but I was happy to work with him with the support of his GP, with whom I could get in touch should it prove necessary. I also had the facility to refer him to a dietician, but his progress was such that this was not needed. He was already on antidepressants which he found helpful, and they could be increased or decreased as appropriate.

There were several things that traditional therapists would have liked to explore, such as the break-up with his girl friend and the death of his father when Vic was 19. I chose to leave these issues alone, thus freeing up time to find solutions to the problem he had come to therapy with.

His bulimia nervosa was such that it reduced his social life and his concentration at work. However, he seemed well motivated to recover and ready to take risks to change. I think he entered therapy in the "determination" phase. I started re-framing his notion of him "being a bulimic". He quickly began to see some exceptions in his behaviour, and accepted that he was not as useless as he had thought.

We challenged his notion that when he was thin he was blissfully happy. This was an anorexic phase, when he exercised compulsively and did not eat much. It led to social isolation which, with the benefit of hindsight, was not attractive at all. It is common for such periods of starvation to turn into compulsive binge eating or bulimic phases. It was a relief for Vic to know that he was not alone, and that he was not going mad.

You may have noticed that I did not respond to his wish to know *why* he had this eating problem. This is because solution-focused therapy is not interested in "how and why" issues, as these explorations make therapy lengthy and depressing. Instead, I asked him to state a more positive goal, which was overcoming his eating disorder so he could lead a more normal life. We deduced what "normal" meant to him from his Miracle Day details.

He did not assume that he needed to be fully recovered in order to finish therapy. He felt that getting to 7 was "good enough". A little work was needed to explain what was meant by small, achievable steps. This is a very important issue in recovery from eating distress as clients often want to leap into health, which for most is just not possible, and failing to achieve unachievable goals leads to another opportunity for self-deprecation.

Session 2

Session starts with the usual greetings.

T: Tell me what has been good since we last met?
V: Not much really.
T: Hmm? [Waits]
V: I suppose I tried what we agreed. I set my alarm half an hour earlier on the day after our first session and managed to get up and have some breakfast.
T: Did you enjoy it?
V: [Flatly] It was good, yeah.
T: What did you have?
V: I made up muesli with cereal flakes, dried fruits and nuts. I had it with skimmed milk. It was nice.
T: Sounds delicious! OK, and then what happened?
V: Like we said, I went to work and didn't stop for chocolate on the way.
T: How did that make you feel?
V: Good on the one hand, because I didn't have to do that. But when I got to work I was gasping for some. But I had decided not to take any loose change for the vending machine.
T: Wow, big decisions. You really wanted to make a go of it. What happened next?
V: I have to say, I borrowed some money to get chocolate.
T: What time was that?
V: I succumbed at about eleven o'clock, just before the tea lady came.
T: So that was quite a triumph then ... having breakfast and waiting until eleven to have a "choc-fix"!

V: I suppose you could say that.... I felt I'd let myself down, though. The day went downhill from then on. Once I had started, I was eating and vomiting all day.

Looking for exceptions
T: All day?
V: Yeah.
T: How do you do that?
V: I binge, vomit, binge, vomit. It just goes on, and on, and on all day long.
T: Even when you are in meetings? Even when you are with other people? Even while you are on the phone? Even when you are at the door doing your bouncer job?
V: [Smiles] No, there are times that I don't.
T: Tell me about the times that you don't.
V: Well, as you say, when I'm doing my bouncer job I can't very well stand there stuffing my face. It wouldn't look good. And I can't escape to the loo either 'cause I can't leave the door.

Starting to externalise the eating disorder
T: So at those times you pull a fast one on your eating disorder, you put yourself in a "safe" environment where binge vomiting is not an option?
V: Yeah ... put it like that, I suppose I do.
T: 'Cause for the same amount of effort you could let your bulimia take the lead. Say, for instance, let it lure you into not going to work in the evening, ringing up saying you are ill, so you can stay at home, binge-vomiting all night?
V: I'd *never* do that. I'd *never* let them down at work.
T: You are a very reliable staff member ...
V: Hmm.
T: So in terms of the nightclub you can give the bulimia an ultimatum. "This is as far as I will go," sort of thing.
V: I suppose I do. Yes! [Smiles]
T: I think it's great that you manage to do that at your evening job. I wonder how you could pull a fast one on your eating disorder in your day job?
V: Well, I tried by not taking any cash with me, but then I gave in and borrowed some off a work mate, and then the whole day fell into ruins.
T: Except for first thing in the morning, when you got up and had breakfast, *and* in the evening when you were ... "bouncing"? [Laughter]
V: Yeah. The rest was rubbish, though. Vomited six times.
T: I wonder if you could tell me ... what does a "good" day look like?

V: A good day is a day where I've not binged and vomited.
T: So let me get this clear.... What we are working towards is a day without binge vomiting, and the way to get there would be by trying to reduce it?
V: Yeah.

Homework
T: I wonder if you would be prepared to try something for me. Some other people I work with have done this too and found it useful.
V: I'll give anything a go.
T: Have a look at this graph. Each day of the week is represented, and the days are divided into morning, afternoon and evening. What I'd like you to do, is to put a tick in the space where you feel you have done yourself justice. Don't bother writing anything if you are not pleased with what you have done.
V: Ok, I'll have a go.
T: The reason for this exercise is that many people think, like you explained earlier, that if they slip just the once, the whole day is ruined, so they might as well carry on binge vomiting. And when they look back on the day they see one huge negative blob, and then they can beat themselves up over that.
V: Exactly.
T: Whereas if we stand back and look critically, we see that there are some aspects that were not bad at all.
V: Like when I'm doing my bouncer job.
T: That's right.
V: Yeah, I'll give it a try.
T: OK. So shall we call this the "homework" for this week? Would you try another "early rise" if you felt so inclined?
V: I think I will give that another go as well.
T: Great. Do you feel we've talked about all the things you wanted to raise today?
V: Yep. This will keep me going.
T: Where do you feel on our scale of 0–10 in terms of overcoming this bulimia?
V: At the end of this session? 2.5.

Compliments
T: I think we've covered quite a lot today. You managed to get up early, and felt the benefit of that. And now you're keen to try some more things to help you conquer the bulimia some more.
V: Yeah ... I seem to be going somewhere at last.
T: That's good. When would you like to meet again?
V: Can we make it in another week? [Appointment is arranged]

T: OK, see you then.

Evaluation of session 2.
Vic shows a common trait found in people suffering eating distress. If the whole day is not perfect, then the whole day is rotten. This black-and-white thinking opens the way to more self-disgust. Clients feel they can't get anything right. They make huge promises that they will never binge vomit again and the next day find themselves at it once more. Splitting the day in three seems to work well for my clients. (I have even worked with a woman who split the day up into hours to begin with.) This proves that huge chunks of the day may have been acceptable or good, and gives clients the opportunity to look at what they do that works, so they can do more of it.

Vic had been able to complete his homework task, and in doing so had started on the way of self-nurturing by preparing a decent breakfast.

Session 3
T: Hi Vic, what's been good this week?
V: Not much, really. I've done my homework. [Gets paper out of pocket]

1	Monday	Tuesday	Wednesday	Thursday	Friday	Saturday	Sunday
Morning		Good			Good		
Afternoon							
Evening	Good	Good			Good	Good	

T: So what do you think?
V: Load of crap.
T: Is it? I don't understand, 'cause I see "Good" so often. Can you explain your "Good" entries?
V: Well, the evenings that were good was when I was at the nightclub. Apart from Monday, that was after I came here and I didn't binge in the evening.
T: Wow. What did you do instead?
V: I had a Weight Watchers' meal and bread, and put all the chocolate in the freezer.
T: Out of temptation's way?
V: Too right! [Laughter] Couldn't touch it then!
T: What impresses me is that you didn't allow your eating disorder to persuade you to defrost some!
V: I'm quite pleased with that, really. But look at this: in the afternoons I've been bad every time. And the mornings are not much better.
T: Tell me about the two good mornings?
V: Well, I managed to get up early and have breakfast. I didn't stop at the petrol station for chocolate and I took a healthy lunch in to work.

T: Wow. How did you motivate yourself to do that?
V: I really wanted to come here with something to show for it.
T: Great. What thoughts went on in your head to support you to do this?
V: I went to bed reasonably early, so I wasn't too knackered in the morning.
T: And because you felt more energetic ...
V: I could get out of bed with time to spare to make lunch.
T: I'm interested to hear what you prepared for your healthy lunch.
V: Two rolls, a yoghurt and some fruit.
T: So you must have gone shopping with "healthy lunch" in mind, to have that sort of food in your cupboard?
V: Funny you should say that. I guess I did 'cause I didn't buy as much chocolate, crisps and biscuits as I usually do.
T: Fantastic! So there you were, having got up earlier, not as knackered, getting to work with a healthy lunch. What happened then?
V: On the first good morning I ate a roll at 11 and then another one half an hour later. Then at lunchtime I bought some food and sicked it up. Then I was sick a few more times.
T: So on Tuesday you were sick considerably less than normal?
V: I suppose three or four times.
T: And then you had a good evening.
V: Yep.
T: Friday was a good morning too. Can you talk me through it?
V: Got up early again. This was really good because I didn't eat both rolls before midday. I kept one for lunchtime. But then I didn't feel I'd had enough, so I bought an egg and cress sandwich and a few bars of chocolate, scoffed the lot and sicked it up. But it was difficult because there were a lot of people and so I couldn't get rid of it all. Which made me frustrated.
T: Very complicated, isn't it.
V: You have to be clever.
T: The eating disorder makes you devious?
V: It does. I know exactly when I can use the loos, but on Friday there were more people around.
T: But altogether a day to be pleased about?
V: Better than the others, anyway.
T: Where do you feel you are on our scale today?
V: Having worked with this schedule this week I think I've gone up half a point.

Homework task
T: So you are at 3....

V: Hmm.
T: I think you've done a great job this week ... so many new insights and achievements. It's great! So what do you think you need to do to crank yourself up the scale a little?
V: I'd like to have another go at this schedule. See what I can do.
T: Do more of what works, eh? Sounds like a good plan. And when would you like to see me again?
V: Have you got a space next week?
A new appointment is arranged.

Evaluation, session 3

Although Vic could not see it at first, he had made tremendous strides forward. He had begun to realise that he could make choices. He went to the supermarket and changed his normal routine of stocking up with crisps and chocolates. He had food in the cupboard to make a healthy lunch. He went to bed early so he would be more energetic in the morning, and he managed to have two "good" mornings in one week. He also began to see some distinct disadvantages to binge vomiting, e.g. on Friday it was difficult because there were more people around. We also re-framed his notion of "being good" and "being bad" to "having a good/bad morning", which separated him from the eating disorder.

Session 4

T: Hi Vic, what's been good this week?
V: I thought you'd ask that question!
T: Beginning to know me, eh?
V: Yep. Uh ... what's been good is that I have had some more good parts in the days. [Shows graph]

2	Monday	Tuesday	Wednesday	Thursday	Friday	Saturday	Sunday
Morning	Good	Good	Good		Good		
Afternoon		Good					
Evening	Good			Good	Good	Good	

T: Tell me about the good times.
V: Well, Monday was last week. It started good because I was coming here and I was motivated. Then in the afternoon, the usual, eat, sick, and the evening was good. But I'm pleased about Tuesday cos I got up early, made lunch and I didn't throw up in the afternoon
T: Tell me more!
V: It wasn't easy. It wasn't easy at all. But I had made my lunch and I bought some extra, but I just decided, I'm just not throwing this up, cos if I do I'll only want more. What a waste of effort! What a waste of money! So although

    I wanted to, I didn't.
T: Wow, fantastic, a breakthrough! And how long were you bothered by the "I must throw up" thoughts?
V: They lasted about an hour.
T: And then?
V: They got a bit less and I got some work done. I felt much better for it.
T: I guess you would feel better. Because you had some decent grub inside you, it was allowed to stay there, and you didn't lose it, plus your stomach juices and electrolytes and what ever else should be swimming around you, down the pan!
V: I know. It's not even that easy, throwing it up. It makes my head throb, it makes my eyes puffy.
T: You are working against gravity when you vomit I suppose. Our bodies are designed to let things go down rather than up.
V: Yes, that's right. Stupid thing to do …
T: So the benefit of not throwing up was that you had more energy to do your work?
V: I think I concentrated a little better, yes.
T: Who noticed?
V: My boss must have noticed because I got a report on his desk on time.
T: And he would be pleased?
V: Yeah, he was pleased.
T: Great … the effort really paid off for you then.
V: Trouble was yesterday. I got up late, had a binge and a vomit, went to my mum's for lunch, ate everything in sight, vomited several times, felt so lousy when I got home that I ate my way through anything I had in my cupboard and threw it all up. I really thought I had it licked on Tuesday … very disappointing.
T: Can I share something with you which some of my clients find useful?
V: Go ahead!
T: Well, most people think of themselves as being the problem. Like you said in the first session, "I am a bulimic." People often describe it as feeling a tension, a tightness, somewhere in their chest.
V: Yeah.
T: Well, what I would like you to try and do is to imagine taking that tightness out of your chest.… And put it on your shoulder. [Demonstrates by pretending to lift something from the chest and put it on the shoulder] This may sound a little strange, but we could look upon your eating disorder like a monster. It sits on your shoulder and relentlessly whispers in your ear: "You're useless, you're good for nothing! Why don't you have something to eat and it

will feel a lot better!"
V: That's right!
T: But basically, all it's doing is feeding you rot. It slowly brainwashes you. All it wants to do is to let you look on the negative side, so you can carry on beating yourself up.
V: I seem to be doing that, all right.
T: It wants you to feel so bad about yourself that you begin to think no one else could possibly like you, so you might as well sit on your own at work, or stay at home, instead of meeting your mates in the pub ...
V: That has been happening a lot ...
T: Whereas what *we* are interested in is, OK, we accept that things aren't absolutely rosy at present.
V: You can say that again! [Laughs]
T: But what are you doing when things are not quite so bad? And how come, when you have slipped, you pick yourself up again and start afresh?
V: I dunno really.
T: OK, let's look at your graph here. We can see straightaway that some progress has been made, because there are nine "good" entries compared with the six last week. But even without this, you are proving that even after a "bad" night, you can turn around and have a "good" morning. *And* you are even managing to have a "good" afternoon!
V: Yeah, I suppose so ...
T: But what your monster wants you to do when you've slipped, is to say, "Oh, go on, I've done it now, let's carry on." And then you can feel even more of a failure, and binge and vomit some more.
V: That's how it goes ...
T: And while you're feeling low, it whispers, "Why don't you eat some more? Go on, it will make you feel better! You can always sick it up again, and then you won't put on any weight!"
V: That's *exactly* how it goes!
T: But between us, we are beginning to rumble your monster. It is telling you a pack of lies. You are bingeing and, granted, maybe you *do* get some pleasure from that, but in the meantime you are telling me that you are putting on weight.
V: Yes, I'm still piling it on. Had to get some bigger trousers at the weekend. Found that really upsetting.
T: So we can deduce that vomiting is maybe not such a useful way to control weight?
V: I suppose it isn't, no. I guess I can't be bringing *everything* up. But what could I do instead?

T: What has worked for you in the past?
V: Swimming, but I can't do that until I'm thinner. I won't be seen dead in trunks at the moment. I'm too fat.
T: OK, so not swimming. Anything else?
V: I'm saving up for an exercise bike. When I'm thinner I could go out and ride a pushbike.
T: So an exercise bike could be an option? How would you go about it?
V: I could start looking at the adverts in the paper, see if I can pick one up second hand.
T: And how likely is it that you will be able to start looking?
V: On your scale? A 10.
T: So we have established that it is time to start looking at alternative forms of weight control. Just for the record, where on the scale do you feel today?
V: I feel at least a 3. I feel motivated to tackle this now. I like the idea that my eating disorder is a monster on my shoulder.
T: Hmm, that's what some of my other clients say too. This means that you no longer have to say, "I am a bulimic." I guess it's kinder to say, "I'm recovering from bulimia."
V: Yeah. [Thinks for a while] Yeah, that makes a big difference.
T: And instead of beating yourself up when things don't go as planned, you could give your monster what-for?
V: [Laughing] Too right I will!
T: And I suppose that if something good happens, you could say, "One in the eye for the eating disorder."
V: Yeah, that's right. To battle!
T: If it has been a good battle between now and when we next meet, where will you be on the scale?
V: I'll leap to a 4, I think!
T: Has this been a useful session today?
V: Very useful. It's good to think that I can fight a monster rather than myself. I'd like to make another appointment but I can't come next week, can we leave it a fortnight?

A new appointment is arranged.

Evaluation of session 4
Vic managed with difficulty to resist the temptation to throw up on Tuesday afternoon. To make it easier for him next time, I asked him for a detailed description of how he did it. We established that the urge to vomit wore off after an hour, which is something I am often told. He then felt better for having eaten and kept it down.

I introduced the externalising idea more fully in this session, feeling that it could help him to begin beating himself up less, which in turn would free up time to work on his recovery. He responded well to the idea that the eating disorder was a monster on his shoulder, it made our work more light-hearted. We established that vomiting was not very effective as a means to reduce weight and explored healthier ways of weight loss.

Session 5

T: Hi, Vic. What has been going well for you these two weeks?
V: I think the first week went well. But the second week wasn't as easy. I wasn't able to get up as early. I don't want to make excuses, but I think it's because I had a bad cold ...
T: OK, let's start with the first week.
V: I have done battle with the monster and I think I've won a few times.
T: Tell me more!
V: When I left here I walked home 'cause my car was being repaired. I walked by the bagel shop. I normally call in there and get two bagels but I imagined the monster being in there, trying to persuade me to go in. So I said "Piss off," and walked straight past!
T: Goodness! How did you do that?
V: I thought about what we'd talked about in here. I thought, "I have some food in the house, why spend money here.... I could save a few quid and put it towards my exercise bike!"
T: Hey, fancy that! How did this make you feel?
V: I have to say I felt good being able to do that. I didn't know I could do that, you know, walk straight past temptation. Thinking of the monster definitely helped.
T: Last time we spoke about exercising, looking for ...
V: [Interrupts] I haven't got a bike yet, but I have started using the car less.
T: Good compromise, I suppose?
V: Yeah, it stops me just sitting around all the time, so now I walk into town and I walk to the nightclub and home again. I didn't walk as much this last week because of my cold. I've brought my schedule....

3	Monday	Tuesday	Wednesday	Thursday	Friday	Saturday	Sunday
Morning	Good	Good	Good	Good	Good	Good	
Afternoon			Good				Good
Evening	Good			Good	Good	Good	

4	Monday	Tuesday	Wednesday	Thursday	Friday	Saturday	Sunday
Morning	Good					Good	
Afternoon			Good				
Evening			Good	Good	Good		Good

T: Talk me through it.
V: Well, I think things were improving. I didn't binge vomit most mornings in the first week. I got up and had a decent breakfast.
T: So the overall picture was pretty good. How do you make this work?
V: I think dividing the day up in three is a breakthrough because I can see that I only have to "keep it going" for a part of the day. It doesn't all murk in together. The monster tries to tell me that just because I've slipped I have to ruin the rest of the day, or the whole week! But I can see now that I'm getting more good mornings.
T: So what's next?
V: Well, I need to get up early again I suppose ... and then I'd like to try and improve on my afternoons. Start walking some more again.
T: I notice you had a good afternoon on Wednesday and Sunday ... and in the second week on Saturday. What happened there?
V: Let me think. Wednesday ... I can't quite remember but I was busy. Must have thought about the monster, not letting it get the better of me. But on Sunday I went to my mum's and I didn't eat too much. It was saying to me, "You're not eating enough, you're not eating enough!" But I said, "I *am*. I'm eating as much as I need and then I'll stop so I don't have to vomit."
T: Crafty things, these monsters, aren't they? When they tell you "You're not eating enough" it means, "You're not eating enough to make yourself sick, so go and have some more and then you can have a jolly good throw up."
V: Yeah, that's exactly how it goes. I'm beginning to understand that now.
T: It went well at your mum's, then?
V: I think so ... I was a bit anxious after lunch, you know, wanting to throw up
T: But you didn't. How come?
V: I told my monster to piss off again, and there was a good film on telly, so it took my mind off it.
T: So what happened was that you did feel the urge to vomit, but then you "put glue on your seat" and stayed put, concentrated on the telly, and the urge to be sick wore off?
V: Yeah.
T: And that's a positive feeling?
V: Yeah. I pulled a fast one on it.
T: Did your mum notice?
V: She didn't say, but we did have a nice chat. I wouldn't normally have done

that because I'm so wrapped up with "food-stuff-binge-puke" going round and round my skull!
T: So because you ate a normal amount you didn't have food-thoughts and instead ...
V: I was able to chat with me mum.
T: Hmm! So, bearing in mind this past week wasn't quite as good, which may have had something to do with your cold ... but we notice the successes that were in there as well. Where would you put yourself on the scale?
V: I think today I'm at 4, I feel I've turned a corner again. I always feel better on the days I come here.

Compliments and homework
T: Great. I think you've done really well this past fortnight, in spite of your cold, and I admire your determination to pick up again. And Sunday afternoon – that can be classed as a triumph!
V: I am well pleased with that, yeah.
T: So what do you need to do to stay at 4, or go up a little, maybe?
V: Fight the monster some more I suppose. Get up early, do more walking, look for an exercise bike.... I'd like to start losing some weight.
T: And how will you do that?
V: Look at what I put in my gob. Exercise more ...
T: So do you think this could keep you busy until we next meet?
V: Should think so!
A new appointment is arranged.

Evaluation, Session 5
This was the first two-week gap in therapy and Vic managed the first week very well. He slipped in the second week, probably due to feeling unwell because of a cold. He had started to make some spontaneous changes, such as walking more often, and had on several occasions resisted temptations of food. He managed himself to devise a plan to "get the show back on the road" and we looked in detail at the successful afternoon he spent at his mother's house.

Session 6
V: Don't even ask what's been good this week. It's been a crap week. I haven't done my schedule ...
T: That's OK. Don't worry.
V: 'Cause it's been crap, crap, crap all week long. The monster has had a field day. I'm not losing any weight. I'm wondering if it's in the genes anyway. My mum's fat, my dad was.... Only slim one is my sister. Maybe I'll just never

lose any weight. [Getting tearful]
T: Sounds like a bad week.
V: Too right it was. Binge, vomit, binge, vomit, binge, vomit. Day in, day out. I've gone right back to 1.
T: [Jokingly] Stop, stop! Did you have time for *anything* else?
V: Not much.
T: Is it useful to tell me about it?
V: Well, it was time for the annual stocktake. Loads of things needed sorting. I thought I could stay on top of it, but then two people went of sick and I ended up doing overtime; had to ring the nightclub to say I couldn't come two evenings …
T: That is difficult for you. I remember you saying you don't let them down.
V: Exactly. So there I was, raiding the vending machine. I must have eaten my way though a whole week's supply for the entire firm! Chocolate, chocolate and more chocolate, washed down with fizzy drinks to make vomiting easier. Disgusting.
T: I was wondering … did you get some comfort out of that?
V: No. None at all. In fact, I think it made me feel worse. But then I would find myself getting more chocolate and borrowing a pound here and a pound there. People must think I'm mad!
T: What I think is admirable, is that you can be so honest about it here. Your eating disorder is not allowed to get you to be secretive about it.
V: I value these sessions. If I couldn't be honest here, I don't think I could get better. [Thinks for a while] And in case you want to know where I am on the scale, I feel at 1. Disgusting.
T: I am impressed that you have not slipped to your lowest point of 0. What stopped you?
V: I don't know. I suppose somewhere I knew that I was very down but it would wear off at some point.
T: And has it?
V: I feel a bit better today. I haven't had as much chocolate …

Teaching
T: So not having as much chocolate makes you feel better?
V: It seems to.
T: There is this theory about chocolate which I'd like to run past you…. See what you make of it. It goes like this. [Draws diagram] At this point, (a), you feel empty, either physically low, simply because you are genuinely hungry, or maybe mentally low. So what do you do to perk yourself up? Have a bar of chocolate! Now chocolate is full of fat and highly refined carbohydrates called glucose. This is a substance

that is very easily absorbed by our body, so it doesn't take long before there is a decent rise in blood sugar and we experience a surge of energy, getting you to (b).

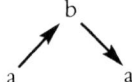

V: That's what I'm after!
T: Yes, but the *nasty* thing is that this energy quickly peters out, and "boing!" down you go, leaving you back at (a), where you started. So what do you do? Have another bar of chocolate! So up goes the energy level to (b), down it crashes again, and what do you do?
V: Sounds familiar. Go to the vending machine and get another bar of chocolate.
T: Hmm. See a pattern emerge here? Up, down. Up, down.... Now, if we consider that chaotic eating causes a chaotic mindset, it is fair to assume that your mood goes up-down, up-down with it!

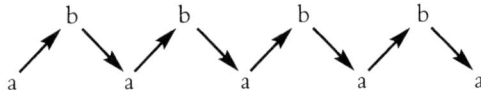

Refined carbohydrate: Quick, short-lived release of energy

T: Does this make sense?
V: Definitely. Uh ... would this be why I can't concentrate at work?
T: I guess it could have something to do with it. The chocolate and the vomiting.
V: So what do I do?
T: Well, we can also look at what happens when you eat something different. Can you give me an example of something you eat that you feel does you justice?
V: It's my breakfast, actually. I make it up myself, like a muesli, with dried fruits and nuts in.
T: Great example. OK, so here we go again. You feel empty; too right you do, it's breakfast time and you haven't had anything to eat for hours! [Laughter] So you decide to eat your muesli. "Aha!" says your digestive system, "Here comes something complicated. We need to chew on this for a while." The chewing motion promotes the production of saliva, a digestive juice, which starts to break down some of the complex carbohydrates in the muesli. The fruit sugars (fructose) are similar to our own blood sugars so they are quickly

released, and absorbed in the blood stream to give you energy. But gastric juices are drawn in to break down other particles further. The pancreas gets alerted: "Send some insulin. We have complex carbohydrates to deal with here!" And slowly, various components are broken down and their energy is released into the blood stream at regular intervals. A nice, gradual process. After a while, when your breakfast has finally left your stomach, you may feel peckish again. What could you eat instead of a chocolate bar?

V: I like bananas.

T: Great choice! They are low in fat, totally natural, contain complex carbohydrates and fructose and they have a minute trace of antidepressant thrown in for good measure! So there you are, munching your way through your banana. The digestive tract follows the same regime as it did for the muesli. You can see on this drawing that we do not have the peaks and troughs caused by refined carbohydrates, which illustrates that ordered eating results in an even mood.

a   b ⟶ a ⟶ b
Complex carbohydrate: Complex carbohydrate:
Slow, gradual release of energy   Slow, gradual release of energy

T: What else do you think would give you the same gradual release of energy as your bowl of muesli?
V: Dunno. [Thinks for a while] Would a roll do it?
T: Would it depend on what you put in it?
V: I could make one with chicken and corn. I like that.
T: Brown or white?
V: They say brown is better for you.
T: Takes longer to digest, releases energy more evenly into blood stream.
V: Makes sense. So what you are saying is, stay away from the chocolate?
T: Do you think that's feasible?
V: Now I know what it does to me, maybe I could eat less of it.
T: Sounds like a good plan. On a scale of 0-10 how likely is it that you will be able to reduce your chocolate intake between now and when we next meet?
V: I'd say quite high, really, 8 or 9 ... maybe even a 10. Reducing it shouldn't be too hard!
T: What we could look at, as well, is what could you eat instead of chocolate?
V: Well, as I say, I like bananas
T: What else?
V: Would cereal bars do?
T: They are full of complex carbohydrates, you could get the variety with dried fruit in it, so they will tide you over nicely. With these new "tools" in your

toolkit, what difference will it make?
V: I'm learning to be more in control. Before I felt useless, but I know that if I can beat this I'll feel better. If I don't eat all that chocolate, I won't have those mood swings. If I eat complex carbohydrates I will have a more even mood. That's got to be worth it!
T: So putting the right fuel in …
V: Yeah, no point putting diesel in the petrol engine! [Laughter]
T: Good way of putting it.
V: I'm gonna give this a go.
T: Look forward to hearing how you got on.
An appointment is arranged for the following week.

Evaluation, session 6

Having done very well to-date, Vic experienced a "dip". This is not at all uncommon, and we simply continued trying to find exceptions. We were concerned about his chocolate intake and looked at the metabolic effects of refined v complex carbohydrates, which he found useful. He decided that he would try to reduce chocolate and thought of better alternatives. He was able to make the link between chaotic eating-chaotic mindset v regular eating-even mood.

Sometimes it is good for clients temporarily to cut out the "trigger food", but this must be done with great care to ensure that it does not lead to malnutrition. I also like to impress that this is a *temporary exclusion*; it is only a means to an end. What we are working towards is a situation where clients can safely include the food again as part of an enjoyable, well-balanced food intake.

Session 7

V: Ask me what's been good this week!
T: Hello, Vic, what's been good this week? [Laughter]
V: I've done what you said. I've reduced my chocolate intake.
T: Impressive. How do you feel?
V: I feel I've cracked it! Every time I reach for my wallet to get to the vending machine, I imagine the monster sitting on top of it, saying "Here, Vic! Come and have a chocolate bar." I can almost see it sitting there. It's the "Choc-Fix Monster", all brown and fat and flabby, and I say, "I know your game, you can bog off. I'll have a cereal bar instead." I feel great!
T: Wow, fantastic! I like your picture of the "Choc-Fix Monster". [Laughter]
V: I've hardly had any chocolate. When I want some I think of the drawing you did last week: up-down, up-down. And I think, stuff that. I don't need that. I got on the scales and I've lost three pounds.
T: Vic, that's fantastic! I just *have* to ask you, where are you on *our* scale today?

V: Well, I'm still vomiting quite a bit, but far less than I used to. So I'd say – ha, ha, I thought you'd ask me this – I'd say a 5 or 6.
T: That's an impressive improvement.
V: Yep. I'm really pleased. And tonight I'm gonna go to see a mate. His wife has an exercise bike but she never uses it, so I'm gonna borrow it and see how I get on.
T: Wow, there's no stopping you now!
V: Good, innit?
T: So tell me again, how has it all happened?
V: Well, when I left here I felt that I understood it all so much more. I knew I was buggering up my system, you know, with all the chocolate. It seemed like an addiction. But then we talked about what it's doing to me … and to my mind … and I don't want to be with my head above the pan all the time. You know, it's stressful, trying to be quiet about it and all that, so others don't hear that I'm in there, throwing up. And I thought, "Blimey, if I can have a whole evening without binge-vomiting at the nightclub, I should be able to do it at other times, shouldn't I?" It all just made sense, you know, all the stuff we talked about, and it all fell into place.
T: Impressive. What can I say?
V: Well, I do want to thank you for being so patient. I couldn't have done it without your help, I have to say
T: Thanks for that. It's great when you see clients switch their light on, when you see them turn a corner. Well done, you have worked so hard you deserve this. Now, what next?
V: I think that if I get this bike home I'll exercise several times a week, and then I hope to see the weight come off. I now have good mornings almost every day.
T: And what's better?
V: I dunno, I jut feel so much better. More confident, more energy. Oh. I haven't brought my schedule.
T: You don't seem to need that at the moment, so …
V: No, I'm getting the hang of it. And at work, I take a packed lunch. I do get chocolate cravings but not as bad.
T: I suppose it's important to have sufficient nutrition each day. You know, so you don't *underfeed* yourself and fall into the anorexic trap again. How will you prevent that?
V: No danger. I have three rolls now, I eat one at 11, so I don't go to the vending machine. Then another one with a banana and a yoghurt at lunch time, then another one in the middle of the afternoon. And I have cereal bars with me so I can nibble on those. I don't go hungry. *And* I've lost a few pounds.

T: Sounds good to me. And no need for choc-fixes?
V: Far less. I seem to have money in my pocket now.
T: And the vomiting?
V: Far less, too. Maybe once or twice a day.
T: So, assuming you get this bike, and exercise … how likely is this to happen?
V: Very likely. If you want me to scale it: At least a 9.
T: OK. And where will that bring you on the "recovery scale"?
V: I think at a steady 6.
T: Looking back over our notes, I see that you wanted to get to 7.
V: Yep. I still need to lose some weight, and vomit less, but I'm getting there.
T: Wow, this is really great. Big grins all round. [Vic grins from ear to ear] So would you like another appointment?
V: Definitely. Can we make one for a fortnight?

Evaluation, session 7

Vic came in to the room triumphant, grinning broadly. The previous session had given him some valuable insights, which had enabled him dramatically to change his eating pattern. From bingeing on chocolate, he now took healthier foods to work, and virtually cut out chocolate consumption. He had visualised and named his monster, which made it easier for him to fight the eating disorder. He also made concrete plans to do more exercise to get his weight down. He was able to see the benefits of eating a regular diet, and had noticed his confidence and energy levels had increased.

Session 8

T: Hi Vic, what has been good since last time? [Laughter]
V: It's been very good. I can't believe it! I've hardly been sick and I've lost another three kilos.
T: So you're really putting your monster to the test here. No vomiting *and* losing weight. You're proving that it *can* be done. Tell me how you're doing it?
V: Well, all my mornings are now good mornings. Except the weekend. If I have a chance I have a lie in. But no binge-vomiting when I get up.
T: Wow! So it still counts as a "good" morning then.
V: Yes.
T: What else is happening?
V: I take my pack-up to work and don't buy *anything* from that wretched vending machine.
T: So the monster is getting pretty miserable.
V: I should say. Miserable and lonely. The worm has turned! [Laughter]
T: What else is going on?

V: As I say, I take good stuff to work, so the temptation is less to vomit and binge. I just stick to what I've brought and I sometimes even leave with some things uneaten.

T: This is getting even better. What else?

V: Well, I have to say … uh … I've got a new girlfriend.

T: Wow. Where did you meet?

V: I have to say, I had seen her a few times at the nightclub. Fancied her, you know? Thought I wouldn't stand a chance, but the other evening she came up to me and asked when my next night off was! And we went out.…

T: We're approaching Miracle Day here, I can feel it in my bones.

V: I think you're right. I hope so.… Anyway, this week-end I'm meeting her family.

T: No flies on you then! [Laughter]

V: No point in hanging about.

T: What I'm wondering is, how will all your newly found skills in monster bashing help you in this situation?

V: I feel much more confident. I've lost nearly 6 kilos, and it's all going off the top of my legs and the waist! 'Cause I've started on the exercise bike.

T: Great. What else will help you?

V: Jane, my girl friend, is ever so supportive. She actually noticed I was losing weight. That feels good. And she said she'd help me. I haven't told her yet that I make myself sick.

T: OK …

V: I'm hardly making myself sick anymore. Sometimes I do it without thinking, you know. Then I get angry with my monster.

T: It lurks there and pounces when you're not looking.

V: Yeah, miserable git. But I don't beat myself up over it. I think, Oh well, put that one down to experience, and move on.

T: Great. No more wallowing. What else is going on?

V: Knowing that if the monster tells me, "You've not eaten enough," it only tries to trap me into eating more and vomiting.

T: So that helps you to stop when you have genuinely had enough?

V: Yep.

T: So you have now learnt to distinguish between being "Vic-full" or "monster-full"?

V: Yeah, and "Vic-full" feels a damn sight better.

T: Well, what can I say? Well done! It feels like you've made such a leap. Where would you pitch yourself on the scale?

V: This last week, what with Jane, and losing weight … I have to say I'm at 7.

T: Well, that's what you were aiming for. And looking back, you are achieving what you wanted to: vomiting less, eating more regularly, less chocolate and so on. I wonder, what have people noticed at work?

V: They have noticed I've lost some weight. They also notice because I'm not always on the scrounge for money. The tea lady's trade has gone down.

T: What about your concentration?

V: I'd say that has improved lots. Even when the boss came down on me last week, like a ton of bricks, I didn't have chocolate! Now before, that would have led me straight into a binge, but I thought that's just what my monster wants me to do, so I won't!

T: What did you do instead?

V: Well, he got the wrong end of the stick anyway, so I let him get on with it. And later in the day I went to see him and explained the situation. And he even apologised!

T: This is a real success story, Vic. You must be duly proud of yourself.

V: I say it again, I couldn't have done it without you.

T: Thanks. Good teamwork, eh? [Laughter] What impresses me about you, though, is that you are so determined to beat this monster. You have had some setbacks, you know, with the cold and work stresses, and it taking a while for you to start losing weight. And the monster was right there to draw you back in. But you said: "No!" Like Harry Enfield! [Laughter] You made a firm stand against it, and you bounced back. That's great.

V: Yeah. Looking at it like that, it has gone well.

T: You have done well.

V: Yeah. I have, haven't I?

T: You jolly well have. "Bullseye!" as you darts players say.

V: One hundred and eighty! [Laughter]

T: So where do we go from here?

V: Well, I said that once I got to 7 I'd finish, but what I'd really like to do is see you, say, in a month, to touch base.

T: Sounds good to me. Meanwhile, what will you do to stay at 7?

V: Carry on as I am, really.

T: Do more of what works.

V: Exactly. And if things work out with Jane, that shouldn't be too difficult.

T: It's good to have an ally.

V: It certainly is.

An appointment is arranged for the next month.

Evaluation, Session 8.

Vic started to reap the benefits from his hard work: his weight was beginning to drop. On top of that he got himself a girlfriend. He stopped using the vending machine at work and was much more confident. Even the thought of meeting Jane's family did not stress him out. It is a real privilege to be alongside clients when they make such dramatic changes in their lives.

We explored the feeling of saturation and he was now able to distinguish between being satisfied and being lured into binge-vomiting. He became much more assertive with his eating disorder, and this oozed into other areas of his life too: he was even able to stand up to his boss and get an apology out of him. We also re-framed his "Things have gone well," to "I have done well," which was part of his being able to "own" his success. We agreed to meet once more.

Final session
(Vic postponed this by a week)
V: Sorry about not being able to come last week. I went away with Jane for a long weekend and didn't get back until late on Monday.
T: Sounds like fun.
V: It's been good. We went to Bruges for the weekend. Had a great time!
T: Wonderful. How have you been? Say on the scale of 0-10?
V: A steady 7 I would say.
T: Well done! That's what you set out to do last time. So how have you done it?
V: Jane has been a great help. We're on a whirlwind romance, I think. She stays at my flat a lot now, and so the evenings are loads better. But even if she's not there I'm OK now. I get on my bike and peddle away, or read my book, or watch a film. I'm hardly ever with my nose in the kitchen.
T: Terrific. What else?
V: Well, as I say, I've really got going with the exercise bike. I use it three times a week. I kill two birds with one stone because I read while I'm biking.
T: Great economy.
V: Yeah, 'cause it can get a bit boring, you know. But Jane has said we'll get a proper bike for my birthday, and then I can start biking around town and into the countryside.
T: Good idea. Will she come too?
V: She already has a bike, so we can go for a bike ride at weekends and stop off and have lunch in a pub.
T: Remember you wanting to be "normal"? Where does that rate on the normal scale?
V: Close to 10!
T: Wow, you have come a long way. Let's just see what you wanted to happen on your Miracle Day. Do you remember?
V: Yeah, I think I'm just about there, really.
T: Let's remind ourselves. [Looks back to notes of first session] You said you

would not be worrying about work when you got up.
V: I worry a lot less. I feel a lot more competent at work now.
T: You would have lost some weight.
V: I've lost over 10 kg.
T: Wow! In spite of the Belgian chocs? How did you manage those?
V: Jane wanted some so I nibbled a few, but that was it. I didn't even *want* more. And I certainly didn't want the monster to get me to put on any weight. We're hoping to go on a beach holiday in six months, so I have to shed a few more pounds.
T: Nice target to set yourself there. OK, you said you'd have regular meals.
V: I do, most of the time. I have breakfast, lunch, evening meal and a few snacks in between.
T: You thought the tea lady and chaps at work would notice a difference.
V: They have. They had a joke about it the other day!
T: Less grumpy, getting more involved with colleagues rather than sitting in isolation at lunchtime?
V: That's all happening
T: Concentrating better at work?
V: Tick!
T: Vomit less?
V: Once, perhaps twice a week.... I've told Jane about it now and that makes it even easier. I think she keeps an eye on me.
T: Enjoy working at the nightclub more?
V: I do. I feel much better there, more confident.
T: Wow, all these achievements. Where would you put yourself on our scale?
V: Definitely at a solid 7.
T: Congratulations. Do you think this is a good time to stop the work we have been doing?
V: I'm happy with that. If I feel myself slipping, can I come back?
T: Definitely. But let's just see what you have in your tool bag to stop yourself from slipping. What has been the most valuable insight you have acquired over the past 3 or 4 months?
V: I think that being aware of the monster helped a lot. And understanding that chocolate is only a quick fix.
T: What else was useful?
V: It helped a lot when you said I was not alone, and I was not going mad. And my weekly charts, they were really useful. They helped me see that even on bad days there would be something good.
T: Any other thoughts?
V: I think that Jane and I can beat it together, and I think that before long I will

get to 8, when I've lost a few more pounds, vomiting even less. That will be great.
T: It will.
V: What I'd also like to do is to come off Prozac.
T: All in good time. It would be worth discussing this with your GP.
V: I have done that, and she suggests keeping on it for a few more months, and then we will review it.
T: Sound like reasonable advice to you?
V: Yep. And if I feel I go down to, say, a 5, and I can't seem to get myself back up …
T: You just swing on by for a top-up session.
V: That's what I was going to say.
T: Well, all I can say is, well done you, good riddance to the choc-fix monster, and now, upwards and onwards.
V: Too right! And thanks again for all you have done.
T: It has been a pleasure.

Evaluation, session 9
Vic maintained his progress. He had become more outward looking and self-confident and was able to enjoy a weekend abroad without any binge-vomiting. He had virtually reached the description of his Miracle Day. We looked at how he would maintain this progress and evaluated our work together, which to me is an illustration that solution-focused therapy can work very well for people in eating distress. In Vic's case there certainly was no need to explore his history, or the possible origins of his problem.

Vic said solution-focused therapy had been "instrumental" to his recovery. The monster talk, explanations of metabolising refined and complex carbohydrates, scaling exercises and dividing the day up into three were especially useful. He felt respected and understood, and therapy had gone at the right pace for him. He rated our work at 8-9.

Update
Two months after our last session, I bumped into Vic in town. He had his girlfriend on his arm and introduced me to her. He spoke very openly about his progress. He had lost another 9 kilos and was engaged to be married. He felt he was at a comfortable 8 on the scale, vomiting only very rarely (maybe once every three weeks). He had bought a bicycle and had cycled to work a few times, and he had to buy several pairs of new trousers as the old ones had started to fall down! I asked for his permission to use his story in this book, and I am grateful to him for agreeing.

Case study 2: "Poison Berries"
Clients: Parents Jane and Rob (also Rosie, age 9, *in absentia*)
Diagnosis/problem: wanting to eat a varied diet and be more relaxed (overcome selective eating and compulsive behaviour)
Referral route: school matron
Setting: my office
Number of sessions: 3 over 6 weeks, with one follow-up after 3 months
Scale at start: 4. Scale at finish: 8. Follow-up: 9

I received a telephone call from Jane, the mother of a nine-year-old, who wanted to know if I would see her daughter to help her overcome fussy eating and anxiety. I suggested seeing the parents first to assess if I would be able to help, but Jane attended on her own as her husband (Rob) had unexpectedly been called away.

Pre-session change
The matron at Rosie's school had suggested Jane contact me because I had helped her daughter overcome bulimia nervosa. This recommendation had made Jane more hopeful and relaxed since making the appointment.

Problem-free talk
This revealed that Rosie, their only child, was a bubbly, intelligent girl who loved riding ponies, liked reading and poetry, had many friends and did well at school. They were a close family who lived in an isolated spot, but Rosie had a few friends nearby.

Problem definition
For a few years Rosie's life had been blighted by anxiety, compulsive behaviour and restrictive eating. She was particularly frightened of berries in the garden, thinking they would fall on her and poison her. She was not able to go within a few yards of a berry bush and would not touch or eat berries of any description. Her eating was restrictive but, as her recent school photograph showed, she was not underweight. Both Rosie and her parents recognised it was time for change.

A family friend suggested therapy in London and the parents attended two appointments together. Jane said she felt crushed after the sessions, thinking she had totally ruined her daughter and all the problems were her fault. She felt it was implied that she was over protective and had spoiled her little girl, and that they both should learn to be firm and stand up to her. Jane and Rob were worried about the suggested approach of weekly, open-ended individual therapy for Rosie, followed by family sessions. And all this after a busy school day and a long journey. They decided to opt out. Jane voiced her concern to the school matron, who had monitored Rosie's food intake for a while, and who subsequently gave Jane my name.

Jane's goal was to support her daughter in gaining more confidence in the garden, with friends and at the dinner table.

The Miracle Day
This consisted of the family having breakfast together. They would then go riding without Rosie worrying that she would die of hypothermia, and instead being able to enjoy the event. She would go to a friend's house for a party, and run freely around the garden, laughing and screaming and having fun, not concerned about the berry bushes. Jane would be able to leave her there, rather than waiting in the car down the lane, and Rosie would not worry at all if mum was a little late picking her up – she'd be too busy playing. The family would enjoy the same food at dinner time, and there would be a relaxed atmosphere in the house. Finally, Rosie would be able to go to sleep peacefully, without worrying that she would certainly die overnight or needing mum to say six times that she promised not to die.

On a scale of 0-10 Jane felt they were at 4, because Rosie was so capable in many areas, and indeed was able to eat a variety of different foods. Jane wanted to get to 8, with Rosie eating a more varied diet, being more relaxed, less intent on getting Jane to repeat affirmations six times, and able to walk straight past a berry bush.

I complimented Jane on her mothering skills. What had she done to produce such a wonderful little individual? What a clever daughter she had, not dying from hypothermia, not dying in the night.... How did she manage that? And what about all those accomplishments: reading, riding, poetry... And how come Rosie managed to eat the various foods she *did* eat?

We agreed that I would work with Rosie "by proxy", that is, through the parents rather than face to face, and I introduced Jane to Rosie's monster. We devised a homework task, which involved telling Rosie about the monster out to mess up her fun, and planning how the three of them could try to outwit it.

Evaluation, session 1
This whole family had been affected by Rosie's difficulty and the parent's self-confidence had been seriously dented by (the way they perceived) the analytic approach in London. Jane was initially taken aback when I gave her compliments on the way she had brought up her daughter, but as I backed each one up with facts, she began to own her successes.

We decided we would not invite Rosie to the sessions as we felt this would put her problem "centre stage". She was coping so well in many areas of her life that the plan was to see if her strength and creativity could be used to pull her out of her restrictive eating and compulsive tendencies. Working with exceptions and externalising Rosie's problem seemed attractive to Jane, and she left equipped with some "monster-bashing homework" for the family to try.

Session 2

I met Rob at the second session but Jane was unable to attend. Rob was very pleased by the change their "monster talk" had made to Rosie. She had drawn a monster on one piece of paper, and a unicorn on another. She decided that if the monster was tricking her into doing something she didn't want to do, she would ask the unicorn for help. She then drew a score board and after one week the score was Monster: 2, Unicorn: 6. She had started eating better at school, and had asked mum to reassure her less at bedtime. I was really impressed and complimented them all on their achievements.

The times the monster did win was when Rob and Rosie were playing in the garden and the ball had gone near a berry bush. This had caused her great anxiety, and they all agreed that it would be good if this could be overcome. In spite of these two incidents they felt they had progressed to 6 on the scale.

By way of homework task I passed on the idea of the "invisible armour" which a lot of my clients find a useful tool. "In the morning, while your monster is still asleep (because we know it's a lazy monster), you quietly put on your invisible armour. But you must keep it a secret, otherwise it will lose its spell and won't work. Now go and see if you can trick the monster. Imagine its face when it thinks you're going to do what it wants you to ... and suddenly you do something totally different." This is followed by "noticing" questions: "Let's pretend we have a video camera, filming you tricking the monster." "What do you see yourself doing differently with this invisible armour on? What do you do instead of being scared? Who notices? What is their reaction?" And so on.

Evaluation, session 2

The family seemed to have taken well to externalisation and Rosie's response was overwhelming. It had put a playful slant on her recovery. I complimented the parents on their success and on their love and care for Rosie and each other, and suggested a new homework task to try. Children as well as adults respond to the invisible armour, and I use it a lot to help clients combat bullying.

Session three

Two weeks later Rob attended on his own because Jane was unwell. He was bowled over by his daughter's success. He had put the idea of the invisible armour to her on the evening after our session and she could hardly wait to try it on to trick the monster. The next day she put it to the test. She walked purposefully under a berry bush with Rob by her side – and did not die.

From then on Rosie progressed in leaps and bounds. She went to bed without fussing, her compulsive traits were greatly reduced, she was more confident with her friends, did not need Jane to be at school ten minutes before leaving time, and

Matron noticed a marked improvement in her food intake. At home she tucked into foods she had avoided before and they had surpassed the Miracle Day picture.

Rob said that there were still some strange idiosyncrasies. For instance, Rosie did not like to go to the loo on her own, but wanted mum or dad to be there with her. I wondered how she coped at school or when she was with friends, which showed up useful exceptions. I jokingly hypothesised that this habit would probably dissipate by the time she was sixteen, and the less fuss was made, the better.

We agreed that Rosie's progress was remarkable, and having reached a steady 8, it would not be necessary for us to meet again.

Evaluation, session 3
Over the years some habits and coping strategies had sneaked into Rosie's life that eventually had grown troublesome. The parents had tried to stop her compulsive behaviour by providing extra reassurance, which in turn had made the need even greater. They could see Rosie getting more distressed and this increased their feelings of inadequacy. Looking for exceptions, externalising the problem, focusing on solutions and giving compliments was the right mixture to propel this family into their preferred future.

Update
Jane made another appointment three months later, to give me an update. Rosie was no longer worried about berries, was able to eat a varied diet that included strawberries, and was far less clingy then before. She had won the prize for poetry writing and reading, and also several rosettes at riding events. She was no longer worried about dying, had started to go to the loo on her own, and played happily at friends' houses while Jane went home to do some work. All this brought them to 9 on the scale.

Asked where Jane would rate solution-focused therapy on a scale of 0-10, with 10 being the most useful it could have been, she put it firmly at 10. She and Rob liked the light, playful nature of our work. They felt they had a narrow escape from weekly problem-focused sessions in London, and that the exception seeking, scales and especially the externalisation, had helped them to support their daughter but had also built up their confidence as parents.

Jane and Rob never mentioned my involvement to Rosie, and orchestrated the whole process in such a natural and relaxed way. It left me in awe of this family. So I asked their permission to share their story with you. I hope you enjoyed reading it as much as I enjoyed working with them.

Case study 3: "Mindful Eating"

Donna (40)
Diagnosis/problem: wanting to increase self-confidence and feel in control around food
Referral route: via dietician
Setting: my office
Number of sessions: 5 over 6 months
Medication: Fluoxetine (Prozac), 40mg/day for the past year
Stated weight at start of therapy: 98 kg. Stated weight at end of therapy: 78 kg
Scale at start: 2-3. Lowest point ever: 0.5. Scale at finish: 7.5
Follow-up six months: 8. Follow-up 12 months: 8

Pre-session change
D: I looked forward to seeing someone who specialises in this sort of thing. The dietician told me about the way you work. It made me feel hopeful and a bit less depressed.

Problem-free talk
D: I'm a kind person, and do as I will be done by. I used to live in France and I enjoyed that. I speak fluent French. I am happily married to John and we have a son, Billy. He is three-and-a-half. My husband was married before and has two adult sons. We get on alright. I like reading, anything and everything. I have a lovely house in beautiful surroundings and like walking in the woods, gardening and looking after the animals (chickens and ducks). I'm having two young German girls to stay for a fortnight soon and I'm really looking forward to that, as I'm surrounded by men!

I'm pleased that I have managed to keep my weight stable for three months. I know I haven't lost any more since I stopped seeing the dietician, but at least I did not put the weight back on that I lost under her guidance. I have not binged on ice cream and have been able to just have two or three biscuits out of a packet. I haven't gone foraging for biscuits for ages.

Problem definition
D: I have very low self-esteem, although I put on a brave front and people don't recognise it in me. I have this weight problem … I pig out. I feel unattractive and self-conscious. I've had several attempts at diets, they always fail. I have seen a psychoanalyst who made me feel worse than I was already, and a hypnotherapist but he was no good, either. I think working with the dietician was good, but I seem to have got stuck.

Miracle Day

D: I don't think of food as I open my eyes.
T: What do you think of instead?
D: I think of the day ahead with Billy. I think of maybe visiting a friend.
T: Who will be the first to notice a miracle has happened?
D: John has already gone to work before I come to in the mornings, so he wouldn't. It would be Billy. He'd say, "Mummy, have you had breakfast yet?" Breakfast would not be a problem on that day. I'd have a cup of coffee and cereal with Billy (I don't normally eat with him) and then we'd feed the animals.
T: If you could see yourself doing this, what would tell you that things are different, that a miracle has happened?
D: We would be walking faster.
T: You are walking faster, and …
D: We'd be laughing and smiling.
T: You are laughing and smiling. What do the ducks notice?
D: That I am able to chuck the food further in the pond! [Laughter]
T: Then what happens?
D: We take the dog for a walk, and we go into the woods.
T: What else?
D: I talk a lot more to Billy.
T: And then what happens?
D: I take him to playgroup at 9.30.
T: You've done all that before 9.30? You are early birds!
D: We are on the Miracle Day! [Laughter]
T: Who notices at playgroup that a miracle has happened to you?
D: Other mums notice.
T: How will they know?
D: My eyes are brighter.
T: What else do they notice? Imagine you are looking at yourself standing in this group of mums. What is different?
D: I am more confident.
T: How do you "do" confident?
D: I don't just drop Billy off and scuttle back to my car.
T: So instead?
D: I stay and chat. I am more upright. There is eye contact. I say more. I laugh and joke with them.
T: What happens next?
D: I go shopping. I buy something bright to wear. Then I go and pick up Billy at 12.30. We have lunch, a picnic in the garden. Then I'll try on my new outfit.

Billy will be surprised. He's only ever seen me wear dowdy colours.

T: Wow. What will he say?

D: "Nice, Mummy!" [Laughs]

T: How does the day develop from there?

D: We will visit some friends. They will be very surprised that I have something bright on. After that, Billy and I go into town and book a trip to France for the family. That will be a miracle. I can't go on holiday at all at the moment.... I feel too frumpy.

T: OK, so book a nice holiday, why not?

D: Then we stop off in the supermarket and I put healthy food in my trolley. I feel good about that. When we get home I am able to keep my food cupboards shut. I am not tempted to eat too much. I cook us some supper from scratch, not a ready-made meal as usual.

T: Paint a picture of your family meal for me.

D: We are all sitting around the table. I have put a tablecloth on the table. We have a jug of fresh water and glasses, and I've put flowers on the table. We eat like the French do, taking a long time, chatting, laughing. Billy's loving it. Everyone enjoys what I've cooked, because it is home made.

T: So you know exactly what's in it.

D: Yeah. It tastes much better when you cook it yourself, doesn't it?

T: Hmm. What happens next?

D: John clears up the kitchen while I put Billy to bed. We have a babysitter and John and I go to the pub for a jolly good natter. Then we go to bed and make mad passionate love. I feel sexy and attractive. And I really fancy John again.

Scales

T: Ok, that sounds like a very positive day. *And* a positive evening! [Laughter] I wonder if we could put this on a scale of 0-10, where 0 represents the worst you could possibly feel, and 10 is the Miracle Day. Where would you say you are now?

D: I'd say a 2-3.

T: What is it that puts you there?

D: I have a lovely husband, and Billy, my home ... I have a good life.... I should be nearer a 10 really.

T: OK. Have you ever been lower than 2-3?

D: I have. The first year after Billy was born I was so close to 0 ... I think a 0.5.

T: What helped you get up to 2-3?

D: John was very supportive. The tablets helped, Billy helped – I should not stay that low for his sake. He motivated me. I had an urge to get better.

T: OK, and if our work were successful, where would it help you to get to on

D: the scale?
D: I'd like to get to 7.
T: Just so we know when you've got there, could you say what will be happening at 7?
D: I'll be so much more confident. [Laughs] I will have lost another 10 kilos. I won't feel hungry, even though I shan't be grazing all the time. I will eat normal food, a sandwich for lunch. No nibbling between meals. I will eat the same as everyone else at supper, rather than lying to them, saying I have already had something or that I am not hungry and then go stuffing my face later. I will have time for John, we will be doing things together. I will occasionally wear bright clothes, like a T-shirt or something. I will be able to buy *one* cake or *one* Twix instead of getting a whole load and eating it all myself. I will also be able to go swimming in our pool.
T: Ok, Donna. Now, you say you are at 2-3 at present … what would need to happen for you to get to a steady 3?
D: I think this session has given me some ideas. I could try and cook some food from scratch when I get home.
T: On a scale of 0-10, how likely is it that you will actually do that before we next meet?
D: 10. I'm sure I can do it. I have to stop off at the supermarket on my way home, so I'll get something decent.
T: What might you cook?
D: I'd like to do a stir-fry and noodles. The boys love Chinese food.
T: Hmm, sounds yummy.
D: They will be pleased. I might lay the table nicely as well.
T: Hmm, great.

Compliments and homework
T: From what you have just told me, I think you're a real fighter. Having tried psychoanalysis and hypnotherapy, it takes guts to come and see yet someone else. But it seems to me that you have hit the floor of my office running. You have already achieved such a lot. Maintaining your weight for three months, cutting down on biscuits … You also have a clear idea of what you could do today to start making a difference. And I liked your clear picture of your Miracle Day. So we can start working towards that in small steps, and I wondered if, between now and when we next meet, you could look out for moments when a little bit of the miracle is happening? Like you suggested, cooking a meal from scratch, laying the table nicely … and really paying attention to the difference this makes. What does it enable you to do differently?

Donna agrees and we arrange to meet the following week.

Evaluation, session 1

Donna wanted to lose weight and increase her self-esteem, and in the first session she gave a clear picture of how she saw her life when her difficulty was overcome. While her obesity was acknowledged, we did not dwell on the negative aspects, and focused on what she wanted to achieve instead.

We obtained rich details of the "confident Donna", and changed her tentative descriptions prefaced by words like "would", "could" and "may" into positive expectations using words like "will", "can" and "shall". She created a homework task which she was determined to achieve and set herself a reasonable point to finish therapy.

Session 2

Donna had a good week. She got on well with her two young German guests and having them to stay opened her eyes to what "normal women" eat. She had watched a video of when she was at her heaviest, which had given her a shock and had made her more determined to lose weight. She had surpassed herself on the homework task, having cooked most meals from scratch, sat down to eat with the family every evening, and laid the table nicely every day. She felt putting flowers, a jug of water and nice glasses on the table made a great difference because it turned ordinary mealtimes into a bit of a celebration. I commented that the skirt she wore had some bright specks in it. She had bought it the day before when she was in town with the German girls, and as far as she was concerned, this was another sign that some small bits of the miracle were happening.

She felt at 4-5 on the scale and was concerned that she did not want to lose momentum after the girls went back to Germany. "I don't want to get up with all good intentions, and then slip and feel I might as well carry on all day because I've smashed the day up anyway." I suggested she split the day into three (see Vic's case study, above), and celebrate the parts when she did herself justice.

I also asked Donna if she knew when a binge was approaching, and she said she could usually feel it coming. I wondered if she would consider asking herself, at the crucial moment as she started reaching for the food, "HALT! Am I Hungry? Angry? Lonely? Tired?"

T: So, say you feel as if that huge magnet in your kitchen is drawing you in … you feel you're about to binge. You're about to be swamped by an "out-of-body" experience. [Laughter] You're about to stuff and there is nothing you can do to stop yourself. At that point see if you can ask, "Am I Hungry? When was the last time I had something decent to eat?" If you haven't had anything for four hours, we can assume that the hunger is genuine. So what

can you choose that in the past has not led into a full-blown binge?
D: A sandwich, or a bowl of soup and bread. It's better to stay away from the chocolate biscuits.
T: OK, so you are hungry and you choose a sandwich, and the binge urge disappears. What do you do next? Remember, you're trying to do yourself justice.
D: Uh ... walk out of the kitchen, take Billy and the dog for a walk.
T: So you take yourself away from the feeding trough; away from temptation?
D: Yeah.
T: That sounds clever. Now, if you establish that you don't feel hungry, then you obviously don't need a sarnie. So you can ask: "Am I *Angry?*" And the answer may well be that you are angry with someone, or with something. Maybe you are even angry with your eating disorder for making your life miserable. So how have you dealt with anger in the past, I mean dealt with it *well?*
D: I don't deal with it at all well. I usually take the blame for everything and then I'll eat.
T: OK, so imagine this is a Miracle Day and you're angry. How do you deal with it?
D: I'd go and tell the person, or if I felt that was too difficult I could talk it over with John.
T: Good plan. What else?
D: Take my mind off it. Let it slide off my back.
T: Like your ducks ... water off a duck's back?
D: [Laughs] Yeah. That's right.
T: So you think, "Is this issue really big enough for me to go into a full-blown binge?"
D: That's right, and put it like that, *nothing* is big enough to throw me into a binge!
T: Too right! Now, if you are not hungry and not angry, you might be *Lonely?*
D: Yeah, I binge the most when I am lonely. Strange really, I push the boys out of the house as quickly as possible, and then I feel lonely, and then I binge.
T: Eating disorders thrive on secrecy and isolation don't they? So how can you prevent yourself from being lonely?
D: Go for a walk with them!
T: Hmm, and how else?
D: Do something. Have a bath, have a swim, ring a friend, read a book to Billy.
T: Great. Now, you know you are not hungry, angry or lonely, but this binge is still tickling you. So you ask, "am I *Tired?* Do I really need to stuff my face here? What else could I do that would make me feel better?"
D: Hmm. I could put my feet up, go to bed early, ask John to take Billy off my hands. I could start some embroidery, I haven't done any for ages! That would

be a good idea, because it would keep my hands busy!
T: Great! See how it works. If you next feel a binge slithering up on you, firmly say HALT! What's going on here? [Laughter]
D: Sounds good. I'll do that!
T: What this is really about, is to change mindless eating into mindful eating. You know, mindless being, "out-of-body experience", stuffing without realising you're doing it, and mindful is enjoying ...
D: [Interrupts] Knowing what you are eating and knowing it is doing you some good.
T: Yeah, maybe you could make a mental note of what goes on when you do a HALT?

We arranged to meet a fortnight later.

Evaluation, session 2

We continued to draw Donna's strengths and successes to the fore, and built new coping strategies, such as the HALT intervention and dividing the day into three. I asked her to differentiate between the moments when she was "mindfully" eating, and when the eating disorder persuaded her to "mindlessly stuff her face". I complimented her on her achievements, going from 2-3 to 4-5 in one week was amazing, and making so much of the Miracle happen was impressive.

Session 3

T: Hi Donna, what's been good since we last met?
D: I had a few wobbly days last week. I don't know why, maybe I was premenstrual, but I've had a few binges. I've also had a falling out with my sister. She's so dominating, and I usually have a binge after I've seen her ...
T: Oh, I see, that's difficult. OK ... but I hear you say, "*last* week". What about the past few days?
D: Oh, it's been better.
T: So you've picked yourself up. OK ... and how did you do that?
D: Well, I thought about what it was like when I had the girls to stay.
T: So you did a bit more of what worked for you, then?
D: Yes, exactly; and I started splitting the day into three, which helped a lot. Not feeling so guilty if I had some chocolate in the morning, because I could start afresh again in the afternoon. And yesterday I had a new houseguest arrive, a young boy this time. A guest in the house definitely helps. I buy different foods. I've bought loads of ingredients to cook with, yesterday we had homemade lasagne.
T: Yum. What else has been good?

D: I eat more fruit. I bought cherries and strawberries and kiwis ... I had forgotten how nice fruit can be. I also made a cake from scratch, *and* managed to just have one small slice, rather than secretly scoffing the lot.
T: That's *fantastic*. How did you do that?
D: Well, I said HALT, actually! [Laughs] In the past I'd tell myself, "I'll make a cake for the boys." But sometimes they never even knew about it because I'd scoffed the lot before they came home. And if I was really bad, I'd bake a cake, eat the whole thing, bake another one, give them some and then scoff what was left. But I didn't need to do that this time ...
T: How come, what made the difference?
D: In fact, I thought of what you'd said about the mindless eating, and I thought: I'll make this a Mindful Cake. I decide to make it, I decide what goes in it, and I decide how much I will have of it. And I did!
T: Well, what can I say? I'm so impressed ... congratulations. How does it make you feel?
D: [Big smile] I feel good actually, I feel really pleased. I know that doing that sort of thing actually makes me feel worse, and I wanted the German lad to have a good time. I wanted to do this for him ... make a cake ... and so I did, and the whole family benefited.
T: What else has been different?
D: I still eat with everyone at the table, we never have our plates perched on our knees in front of the telly anymore. You know, about mindless eating? I think I do that in front of the TV. At the table I am much more aware of what I put into my mouth. I know better when I've had enough and because all the others are there, I'm not tempted to keep stuffing.
T: That's great.
D: We stay at the table longer, talking, having a drink ... In the past I would prepare something for the boys and I would read the newspaper. Then they'd go out to play football or feed the animals. And I would pig out. Shameful behaviour, isn't it?
T: It sounds like you didn't enjoy it that much. [Laughter] Where would that have featured on your scale of 0-10?
D: About a 0.5.
T: And now?
D: Oh, being able to eat with them, chat, linger, enjoy myself ... easily at 6-7!
T: What a leap! So tell me again, how did you move from 0.5 to 6-7?
D: Having guests helped. And I think I'm beginning to allow myself to enjoy things. Making meals from scratch, like we said before. You know what you put into the pot! That makes me feel like I'm in charge more. I sit down and have a nice lunch, a sandwich and a salad. I eat so well that I don't feel hungry

between meals so I nibble less ... and the good thing is, that I've lost a few pounds.

Evaluation, session 3
Donna's improvement was impressive. She had a few "low points". We did not go into the "whys and wherefores" of these. Although her difficulties with her sister were acknowledged with empathy ("Oh, I see. That's difficult."), we did not waste valuable time addressing them. This is a very directional approach, which actively leads clients away from the times they feel inadequate. Clients have shown me that as they get assertive with their eating disorder, this assertiveness gets used in other areas too. As therapy developed, Donna gave several examples of times she had been able to stand up for herself, and she began to feel more on a par with her sister.

We looked at how she had managed to pick herself up to 6-7. She was steadily transforming her life, making choices, changing habits, beginning to enjoy life much more. I have the privilege to be alongside these clients when they share their experiences, and it is awesome seeing them come in oppressed and then blossom, as they free themselves from the stifling grip of their eating disorder.

Session 4 *(Three weeks later)*
Donna continued to improve. She had started to walk more and she had invited some friends over with their children. A huge breakthrough was that she was now able to join them in the swimming pool, where before she had been too self-conscious. "I would not go in for love or money. No one was allowed to see me in my swimming costume. I'd pretend to have a sore throat, or a period, or thrush rather than join them in the water." Billy thought it was wonderful, having a splash with his mum.
T: That is a massive turn-around. How did this come about?
D: Well, I remember us talking about losing weight: doing nothing but focusing on the weight and mistakenly thinking that weight loss alone would bring you happiness. And I had a long, hard think about my life. The good things that I have and how my fat has stopped me enjoying it. And I thought, I must start *today*. I'm blowed if I lose any more time with my boys ... so I went and bought this costume. I look quite good in it really, I've lost a few more pounds ...
T: Fantastic. What else has been good?
D: I've been to London for a wedding. There was a buffet and I didn't keep picking.
T: Going from strength to strength. How?
D: [Imitating me] Did I *do* that? [Laughter]
T: You take the words out of my mouth.
D: I knew when I felt full. That's a new one on me. I am now able to tell when

I've had enough and then I say STOP! *HALT!* [Laughter] But what I can't wait to tell you is, I've booked a holiday.
T: Wow. Where are you off to?
D: We are going to France, to see the people I used to live with. I'm so excited. I never thought I'd do that this year.
T: Where on the scale does that bring you?
D: I thought about that. I still have the odd binge, but I can stop it now.
T: Tell me how you do that?
D: I bought a box of choc-ices the other day. I thought, Good, there are four ... one each if we are all there. But then I started on them, and I ate two. But then I stopped.
T: That is just so fantastic, it almost shows more strength than not having any at all. How did you stop mid-binge?
D: I thought, I have a choice here. Either stop now and feel reasonable or carry on and feel terrible.
T: So you stopped. And you felt ...?
D: Well, reasonable. [Laughter] Because it could have been so much worse.
T: What else is better?
D: I'm wearing some brighter colours ... had some jade green on. My relationship with John is improving, I think I'm beginning to feel more sexy.
T: That must please him.
D: It does.
T: And you.
D: [Laughter] Definitely!
D: I am getting braver in the car, I'm driving to places I've never been before.
T: So benefits all round, then?
D: Yeah, it's amazing. Now I binge less, I have more time for other things. I feel so much happier in myself.
T: Well, I must say, it all looks very good indeed. I'm just comparing you as you are today, with what you were hoping to achieve.
D: I must nearly be there. A 7 I'd say.
T: You are. So what tools do you have in your toolkit that will help you stay at 7?
D: I've learnt so much lately. I think regular meals, not beating myself up so much when I slip, making choices, you know, between mindless and mindful eating ... thinking about what I could be doing instead of bingeing.
T: And say a bit of stress comes along, trying to get you to have a mindless binge?
D: I'll say HALT!
T: OK, that'll learn-it. [Laughter] And with your holiday in mind, what will you

be able to do to make things easy for yourself in France?

D: I'm really looking forward to it. I know it won't be too difficult because I will be with John and Billy all the time, so I won't have much opportunity for secret bingeing. It will just be so lovely to see my old friends again, and I feel so much better about myself now. I know I'll be able to enjoy it.

T: Great. I'm just thinking about the work we've done.... What has been a useful tool that you will remember? Something to pack in your suitcase for France?

D: I think the scales are very useful. Because I can see where I am and if I slip, I can think, How can I move up from here?

T: Hmm. Having accomplished so much in such a short time, do you feel you need to see me again?

D: I was thinking about that as I drove here, and I wondered if I could come once more, after my holiday in four weeks' time?

Another appointment is arranged

Evaluation, session 4

Donna showed consistent progress and had reached the "maintenance phase". We reiterated what she had achieved and looked at how she could overcome possible setbacks.

Session 5

Donna returned from holiday full of beans. She had managed to lose some more weight, enjoyed seeing her old friends and felt closer to John and Billy than ever before. She still had the occasional binge but these were becoming smaller and shorter. She felt more energetic, doing things she had not been able to do before, such as going out to quiz nights and eating meals with friends. Her self-confidence had increased and she was even wearing a peach coloured T-shirt. The increased assertiveness towards her eating disorder had trickled over to her relationship with her siblings, who had started to show her more respect. Significantly, while on holiday, she had bought herself some jewellery, something she would never have thought of a few months ago, and a sure sign that she was beginning to like herself more. She finished therapy at 7.5, having achieved what she set out to do; spending less time bingeing gave her more time to enjoy life.

Donna rated our work at 9 to 10, saying that she had felt understood and respected. Her previous experiences had made her feel inadequate whereas after solution-focused sessions she felt boosted and "ready for anything". She found the Miracle Day exercise a revelation, it made her realise she had "stuffed myself in a damp, dark cupboard for far too long and it was time to get out there and enjoy the life that was going on around me." She felt that although she was by no means at her target weight, she was happier now than she had imagined she ever could be, and put this down to the solution-focused approach which she found empowering and uplifting.

Case study 4: "Fun Run"
Neil (35)
Diagnosis/problem: wanting to relax more (and stop obsessive exercising)
Referral route: GP
Setting: GP surgery
Number of sessions: 1
Medication: nil
Stated weight at start of therapy: 65 kilograms
Scale at start: 3/4. Lowest point ever: -1. Scale at finish: 6.
Follow-up 6 months: 7-8

Pre-session change
Calmer. Simply thinking he is going to tackle the problem made him feel a bit more relaxed.

Problem-free talk
N: I lead my own design team at a fairly large local computer firm. I am a hard taskmaster, I work hard and I play hard. I run a lot, marathons and triathlons. I used to run a lot more but I'm not able to do as much at the moment. I just don't feel up to it. That's why I'm here.
T: Is it OK if we discuss what brought you here in a moment? I'd first like to know a bit more about who you are, what makes you tick.
N: Oh, alright, where was I? I'm happily married (five years) and we do not have children. My wife is very career minded too. I like reading and travelling, both for business and pleasure. I am very focused and I write lists so I can keep an eye on what I have done and what is yet to be done. I like to have things planned. I like to know exactly where I stand. For instance, I know to the last penny how much money is in the bank account.

Problem definition:
N: I suppose I am a bit of an obsessive. I have felt "down" for the past two years. I fell to pieces a year ago, and had to have medication. The worst of it was, that I just could not exercise. That made me feel trapped. After a bit I started to feel fine again so I came off the tablets and started back on my usual training regime. But then, over Christmas I had a "black period". Suddenly, out of the blue, for no apparent reason. All I wanted to do was to sit and cry. I felt so

useless. I kept thinking, "Come on, pull yourself together! Don't be such a wimp. Why don't you just go out for a run and get yourself over this?" I like to train on average four hours a day but I just couldn't get myself to do it. Useless!
T: Sounds bad.
N: It was. I sunk deeper and deeper ... started feeling suicidal. It lasted three or four days. That scared me, so my wife made me an appointment to see the doctor. I thought he'd give me some pills again, but he suggested I make an appointment with you. In a way I was pleased because I don't like taking pills. I think they might make me feel even worse, make me lose my sharp edge or something.
T: So if our work is successful, what difference will it make?
N: I'd like to understand myself more. I'd like to feel normal again. I need to find ways to relax a bit more.
T: OK, just to help me get a handle on all this, could you answer a question for me?
N: OK, go ahead.
T: Imagine you go to bed tonight and while you are sleeping a miracle happens and your problems have been resolved. You wake up the next morning, not realising this has happened. What will be the first thing that tells you a miracle has occurred?
N: I don't know. [Sighs and shakes head] I just don't know.
T: [Waits patiently]
N: I guess ... hmm, I guess I wouldn't feel the need to jump out of bed to go running. [Looks surprised as he says this]
T: Hmm. And how does that feel?
N: That feels weird. I never feel like that. Either I get up and go running, or if I don't, I feel guilty that I'm *not* out running!
T: So there you are, just woken up and you're not feeling guilty. What do you feel instead?
N: I don't know. Hmm. What do I feel when I don't feel guilty? It's pathetic isn't it? I just don't know.
T: What would you *like* to feel instead?
N: I'd like to feel relaxed, happy to just lie there.
T: So we have this picture of you lying in bed, just woken up, relaxed, happy.... Who is the first to notice?
N: Suzie, my wife
T: What does she notice?
N: That I'm still in bed. [Laughter]
T: How does she react?

N: She is pleased. She often complains that we never have a chance to cuddle, because I'm always on the move. She says she can't catch me. [Laughter].
T: What happens next?
N: We have a cuddle and have breakfast together.
T: What else is different on this day?
N: Us having breakfast together is a miracle in itself. [Laughter] We never do, because I'm out running so she has breakfast on her own.
T: So what's it like? Describe it to me.
N: It's nice. I can have cereal and toast and not worry about eating too much. We chat, maybe even read the paper. Then we shower, get dressed, and off to work.
T: What do your colleagues notice?
N: They notice I look better, that I'm more relaxed. I can cope with the workload better. I feel more creative.
T: How do you "do" relaxed?
N: The frown has gone, shoulders less hunched.
T: So if the frown is gone, what's there instead? And if your shoulders aren't hunched…?
N: Uh, I'll have a smile on my face and stand upright. I'd be more friendly towards them.
T: They *would* notice a difference then.
N: [Laughter] Yeah.
T: And then what happens?
N: It must be nearly lunchtime.
T: OK, and what else do you do to make this a Miracle Day?
N: Instead of swimming a few quick lengths at Crown Pools I meet some friends for lunch in town.
T: What do they notice?
N: That I prefer the taste of beer above the taste of chlorine in the pool. [Laughter] We have lunch, catch up with all the news and I go back to work.
T: How does the rest of the day develop?
N: Finish work, go home, go for a run with the dog.
T: Is that different on the Miracle Day?
N: Hmm, maybe I won't run as far as I normally do, but I'd still like to get some exercise in.
T: But this time you feel differently about it?
N: There is a difference. Exactly. *I* am in control and enjoying it rather than feeling I *have* to do it and feeling numbed.

Scaling

T: Right, now if we assume that 0 on this scale represents the worst things could ever be, and 10 is your Miracle Day, then where would you pitch yourself now?
N: At this moment? Uh, talking about this miracle has made me feel good actually, so at this precise moment I'd say I feel at 6.
T: have you been lower on the scale?
N: I have. When I had my "black days" I felt −1.
T: And that was around Christmas, you say?
N: Yes, it was scary.
T: I can imagine. Now, what I would like to know is this: How have you managed to turn things around in just two weeks? From being down here to getting to a 6?
N: Well, when I felt so bad, I cried a lot. That helped me a bit, I think. My wife was really supportive. Then I saw the doctor, and talking to him helped me to see that I was not going mad. And after I saw him I wrote a list of things to do. I arranged to have a health check and had a talk with my boss to arrange some time off. I read a good book and I talked loads with my wife and some friends. I phoned an old college friend. Having a long talk with him helped because he had been through something similar himself.
T: Terrific, you set up a good support structure for yourself. Now, where on this scale do you want to get to?
N: I want to be somewhere around 8.
T: What will be happening then?
N: I will have energy on waking. I will occasionally go for a jog, but won't have to every day. I'll look forward to the day and can have a lie-in at the weekend. I'll be able to relax more.
T: So, suppose you were looking at yourself relaxing ... what do you see yourself doing?
N: As I say, able to have a lie-in at the weekend. Able to put my feet up, see some friends for a meal. And when my wife and I work in the garden I'll be able to pace myself.
T: How do you do that?
N: Not needing to have the whole lot done in one day.
T: So what do you do instead?
N: Take it more easy. I could look for smaller projects to do and stop when they are finished. But I find it so difficult, because I like to keep going all the time, otherwise I feel guilty.
T: Mmmm. I'm a bit confused about what you've just said: on the one hand you "like to keep going"; on the other you "want to relax".

N: I don't quite know how to stop myself.
T: I may be wrong here – so correct me if I am – but it seems to me that you have been fighting against yourself for quite a while?
N: I suppose I have. I think you're right.
T: It's just that, looking over the notes I jotted down earlier, you said, "*All I wanted to do was to sit and cry. I felt so useless. I kept thinking, 'Come on, pull yourself together! Don't be such a wimp. Why don't you just go out for a run and get yourself over this?'*"
N: It's awful!

Externalisation

T Some of my clients who have similar problems say that it's like there is a monster egging you on.
N: That's exactly how it feels.
T: *You* knew that you needed a rest, yet your "monster" egged you on, saying, "Don't be a wimp. Pull yourself together!"
N: It did.
T: So what do you want to tell your monster?
N: I'd like to tell it to naff off and leave me alone.
T: In other words, you can get angry with the monster and start being kind to yourself?
N: Sounds like a good idea.
T: So when it's naffed off, what do you do?
N: Then I can relax.
T: So do you think it is possible to tell it to leave you alone so you can relax?
N: I suppose so.
T: So have I got this right: when you feel an urge to exercise, or push yourself to the limit …
N: I could tell it to pack its bags and get on with some serious relaxation. [Laughter]
T: Like what?
N: Like having that lie-in.
T: Suzie will be pleased.
N: That'll be a bonus. [Laughter]
T: So I guess we've unmasked the monster here, that has driven you into relentless exercising, making you think it would make you feel better, but in reality systematically burning you out?
N: Yeah … that's right.
T: And instead of you "mindfully jogging", that is, really enjoying it and feeling the full benefit, it stole the enjoyment and made it a "mindless" exercise.

N: Yeah, no fun at all. I'd like to go for a fun run with the dog again. He'd appreciate it. [Laughter] I think I have a monster at the office too. I know I need to relax more there, I need to take more days off.
T: What will you do to keep them monster-free?
N: Yeah ... mustn't use those days for exercise I suppose. I know, I'll get Suzie on to it – arrange a weekend away or something.

Homework task
T: So in practical terms, what will you be able to do to inch towards the 8?
N: You've given me some very useful insights. It has been good to get a clear overview of what is going on. I suppose I could do a fun run with the dog tonight. Start as I mean to go on.
T: On a scale of 0-10, how likely is it that you will be able to do that?
N: 15. [Laughter]

Compliments
T: Thinking about the things you have told me today, I can see that you are very thorough. You like to give things your very best, and if a job is worth doing, it's worth doing well. What impressed me most was that, when you slipped down to that very scary point of -1, you managed to draw on support to help you out of that dark place. Often people are ashamed and they isolate themselves, but you did the opposite: you talked to your wife, your GP, your friends – you even found a soul-mate to talk things through with. And now you want to give the same care and attention to getting over this difficult time. You recognised that if you work hard and play hard and don't relax in-between, you end up between a rock and a hard place.
N: Too right I did.
T: So now you are systematically putting support in place to get yourself up again, and even in this session you say you've gained insights that helped you look at things differently.
N: Yes. Very useful.
T: So you are now at 6. I wonder, where do you want to take our work from here?
N: I know I am allowed four sessions here, but I feel so buoyed up, I don't think I need to come anymore. I'm just a bit worried that I might slip again, though.
T: Bearing the scale in mind, say you begin to slip from a 6: what can you do?
N: Look at how I got up before, considering taking things a bit easy, boxing the monster off its perch. [Laughter] I suppose that will be OK, and if I need to, can I make another appointment?
T: Sure. So could I just ask what in particular has been useful to you in this hour?

N: The whole experience really, I've never had anything like this before. I thought when the doctor suggested it, that I might be a bit mad to need someone like you. I thought you'd make me lie down on a couch and we'd go over my past and my childhood, and I would cry a lot. So this is a bit surprising really, to have "therapy" [Pulls serious face] that makes you feel good. [Laughter]

T: Great. So what in particular do you think you'll remember?

N: The monster, for definite. Have to get my boxing gloves out. [Laughter] And your scales, they are a good tool. And realising that I am doing things to get myself back on the rails – that's a relief. Knowing that I'm not going mad. And really looking at my training regime. I can see that it has been stealing time from me and from my wife as well. There are things out there that I'd rather be doing.

Evaluation

Nigel came to see me because he had a "scary experience" over the Christmas holiday, when he had felt depressed and out of control. I empathised with the intensity of his feelings and began the solution-focused exploration, which revealed that Nigel was exercising compulsively in line with the condition called athletica nervosa. He relentlessly put his body through exercise regimes, training on average four hours a day. He also had a demanding job which took him abroad on occasions. He looked lean but tired and was not feeling the benefit of exercise anymore. We discovered that he had been in the process of burning himself out, exercising at the expense of his marriage, health, job and social life. The Miracle Question brought to light how he wanted to live his life instead. He responded well to externalisation, which we used so he could start beating up his monster instead of himself, which would in turn give him a chance to relax and pace himself. We also used the scale to mark out where he had been, emphasize what he had done already to get himself better, and decide what still needed to be done in small, achievable steps. He felt that one therapy session would suffice and we agreed I would follow up after six months.

Follow-up

I telephoned Neil six months after the session. I am always particularly curious to see the outcome from "single session therapy".

He said that he had continued to make progress. He was exercising less but enjoying it more, had taken regular days off work to spend time with his wife, when they would go walking, to a show or gallery in London, or just "potter around in the garden". Their social life had improved, they were seeing many more friends for a drink or a meal. The best news of all was that they were expecting a baby – the ultimate proof that he was taking time to cuddle his wife!

He had taken on board the "scaling exercise" and still regularly had to beat the monster off his shoulder, but all in all felt that he had reached a steady 7-8.

Case study 5: "Jump for Joy"
Emily (13)
Problem/Diagnosis: wanting to put on some weight and be stronger (overcome anorexia nervosa)
Referral route: GP
Setting: GP surgery
Number of sessions: 6 over 5 months
Medication: Nil
BMI at start of therapy: 17. BMI at end of therapy: 19.5
Scale at start: 2. Lowest point ever: 0. Scale at finish: 8/9
Follow-up 3 months: 9. Follow-up 9 months: 9

Emily came to see me on her own for the first session. She said her mother had wanted to come, but Emily had asked her not to.

She had not noticed a *pre-session change,* and *problem-free talk* revealed that she liked swimming, being with friends and playing the keyboard. She was in year nine at high school, where she had many friends who were very supportive. At school she enjoyed music and musical history best, especially because they were learning to play African drums. She got on reasonably well with her teachers. Her parents and brother, aged 16, were OK but got on her nerves sometimes. She liked going out with friends but in the past year had been very tired, so after her daily paper round she'd collapse in a heap at home rather than going out to play. She had two cats called Mork and Mindy.

Problem definition
Emily was worried about her low weight (36 kg), and her poor health. For a year she had eaten little breakfast, no lunch and a small dinner, and had steadily lost a quarter of her initial body weight. She was thinking about food all the time, yet did not want to eat. She was bullied at school, and had thought that if she got smaller, the bullies would notice her less. But she had found the opposite to be true. She now thought that their name calling would diminish as she grew stronger.

Miracle Question.
T: What will be the first thing you notice?
E: I wake up. I have a smile on my face, a great big smile.
T: Right, and what else?
E: And I have energy!
T: Hmm. And what will that help you do?

E: I jump for joy. I run downstairs and tell mum.
T: What does she notice?
E: That I'm up early She hasn't had to drag me out of bed. [Laughter]
T: What will her reaction be?
E: She doesn't have to be annoyed with me.
T: So instead she is …
E: Happy.
T: Hmm. Who else notices?
E: No one. My brother is still in bed and my dad has gone to work.
T: What about Mork and Mindy? What do they notice?
E: They see me being happy, smiling … I will be stroking them, making a fuss of them. They liked being played with, with a little mouse they have.
T: So you are happy, mum is happy, the cats are happy. [Laughter] What do you do next?
E: I have a quick wash.
T: Anything different there?
E: I can be quick about it. I notice that my arms have fleshed out a bit.
T: And then?
E: I get dressed, my uniform fits me properly. Then I go back downstairs. My mum notices I have put on some weight. She sees me having some breakfast.
T: Anything different about that on the Miracle Day?
E: It tastes better. It's less of a struggle. I'm not complaining. That will make mum less grumpy.
T: So she is more …
E: Happier, she jumps around. [Laughter]
T: Imagine you're going to school. What will be different?
E: My friends notice I'm a bit bigger, and a bit happier.
T: How do they see that you're happier?
E: I'm laughing, smiling, joking. And eating a lot. I'm more confident.
T: What will tell you that you're more confident?
E: The bullies don't have an effect anymore.
T: Wow! You're able to deal with them, eh? How come?
E: They don't have to pick on me anymore, because I'm a bit bigger and stronger. I stand up to them. I say, "Go pick on someone else!"
T: That will show 'em.
E: Yeah … too right. [Laughter]
T: Will your teachers notice a difference?
E: They will notice I'm a bit more noisy. I can do my work properly, I can concentrate, and don't make mistakes. My PE teacher will notice that I can run faster, and I can hit a ball properly. I have more energy.

T: What happens at lunch time?
E: I go and sit with my friends.
T: What do you do on the Miracle Day?
E: I eat my dinner.
T: What do you have?
E: I have sandwiches, a cake and some crisps.
T: Do you enjoy it?
E: On Miracle Day I will.
T: What else do you do?
E: I play football, have fun, play with my mates.
T: What happens in the afternoon?
E: I'm less tired. I walk home very slowly with my mates, chatting, laughing.
T: And then?
E: I do my paper round. I have more energy for that. Then I go home and have my tea. I eat loads more than normal, which will make my mum happy. My dad notices that, too, and he is pleased.
T: Great. So everyone is having a good time by the sound of it. What is next?
E: I go out, meet my mates in the park. I play some more football and we do a man- hunt in the woods. I'll go home at eight-thirty.
T: Then what happens?
E: I have some cake and some chocolate and a cup of tea. I watch some TV and go to bed.

Scaling

On the scale of 0-10, where 0 represented the worst Emily had ever felt or possibly could feel, and 10 was the Miracle Day, she described having felt at 0 a few months earlier. She was being bullied, feeling very depressed, trying not to eat at all, and not concentrating at school. But today she was at 2: still depressed, still being bullied, but eating a little for breakfast and dinner. Occasionally she could even have lunch. Emily got to 2 with the support of her friends, who encouraged her to eat, and although her parents got on her nerves, she felt they did love and support her. She wanted to get to 8, where she would be able eat normally again (three meals a day and snacks in-between) which would give her more energy. She would have put on some weight, have restarted her periods, and be strong enough to stand up to the bullies. She would be concentrating better at school and have more fun with her friends.

Homework task

We considered what Emily would need to do in order to move up to 3 on the scale, and she identified that eating something at lunch time would benefit her. She said that she didn't have time to eat at lunch time, and anyway, nothing tasted nice anymore. I explained that anorexia "flattens" our tastebuds and they need to be "tickled" by something tasty to wake them up again. How could she do that? We considered the benefits of having several chocolate bars, and she decided that this might not be a good plan as she would feel sick, and anyway, Mum wouldn't let her. So she opted for a cereal bar instead.

Compliments
I thought that Emily was incredibly brave coming to see me on her own, and complimented her on how she had coped to date. I was particularly impressed with how she had managed to get from 0 to 2 on the scale, and by the way she described her Miracle Day. I could see that she was systematic, which would help her move up the scale in small, achievable steps. She also gave strong signs that she had had enough of feeling weak and being bullied, and that she was ready to stand up for herself.

Evaluation, session 1
Emily was obviously in the grips of anorexia nervosa. She recognised the problem and was willing to change. Because of her age and severity of her condition I spoke to Emily's mother and wrote to her GP.

"I saw Emily this morning, and agree with your diagnosis of anorexia nervosa. She has lost weight over the past year, her menses have stopped and she is very food focused. She is unhappy with the weight loss and resulting lack of energy, and is well-motivated to overcome this. We have started to devise a sensible eating plan. We agreed to meet again in a fortnight and I hope her mother will attend so we can discuss Emily's progress together. I am happy to see her on a regular basis and would like her to be weighed fortnightly by the practice nurse so we can keep an eye on her BMI. If I have any concerns I will liaise with you so we can consider alternative treatment. I told Emily about the Eating Disorders Recovery Group and she is considering coming along to that with her mother."

Emily started seeing me on the verge of needing in-patient treatment. When weight drops to this extent the situation can quickly get out of hand, so regular weighing is an important part of treatment. In an ideal world she would have seen a specialist dietician alongside a therapist, but with no such person available on the NHS, I decided to liaise with her GP and her mother, and closely monitored her progress. She was in the determination phase, showing a strong wish to change, with a realistic response to the Miracle Question which indicated that it was fair to expect a rapid improvement.

Session 2
Emily brought her mother, Sally, and we discussed what she would like to see as a result of therapy. Sally wanted Emily to put on some weight, to have her periods back and to be more energetic. Emily reported that she had eaten a cereal bar every lunch

time and that she wanted to eat more to increase her energy. Sally was concerned about Emily's food restriction ("She doesn't seem to like anything. She doesn't eat anything these days"). Sally felt that when she tried to tempt her with "nice new foods" Emily would refuse to eat them, which in turn upset mum.

We found that Emily's palate could in fact handle a reasonable variety anyway: in the last month she had eaten small quantities of chips, burgers, sausages, crispy chicken, baked beans and runner beans, carrots, mashed potato, spaghetti Bolognese, yoghurt, ice cream, gateaux, crisps, nuts, cereal bars, chocolate, choc-chip biscuits, milk shakes, tea, orange juice, Frusibin (a high energy drink), bananas and apples. Therefore, introducing new things might not be necessary.

Emily considered what a "good day" would look like in terms of food:
Breakfast: orange juice and cereal
Mid-morning: banana or apple
Lunch: Frusibin, roll, cake
Mid-afternoon: cereal bar or chocolate bar
Supper: Chicken, mashed potato and carrots
Bed time: tea and biscuits.

On a scale of 0-10, Emily's motivation to do the "morning part" of this day this for three days was 10. She would then see if she could expand on it. Sally felt a lot happier knowing that she could avoid daily struggles around food by giving Emily foods from the "I Like This" list.

Evaluation, session 2

It was good to have an opportunity to enlist Sally's help in Emily's recovery. We managed to iron out some frustrations and found ways of co-operating that would avoid future ructions.

A common point of friction stems from a mother trying to show a child love by tempting her with nice little titbits. It is crushing to have these thrown back at you (sometimes literally) when you have put in all that time and effort. It is useful to establish what the child *will* eat and from that safe basis slowly to start increasing the choices.

Emily remained motivated and came up with some solid, achievable steps to continue her improvements. We arranged to meet in three weeks' time and for Emily to visit the practice nurse after a fortnight. They were welcome to telephone me in the meantime, if they had any worries.

Session 3

Although Sally was invited to attend, Emily said she preferred coming on her own, and asked me to telephone her mum to give her an update after the session. Emily' weight had increased by two kilos in one month. She had toast and cereal every day for breakfast and a roll and cake for lunch. In the shorter breaks she nibbled on cereal bars. This had given her a bit more energy. The evenings were a little more problematic, and we considered what would make them easier. She felt she could eat better if she was distracted, for instance when she had friends to tea or if they all sat at the table for a family meal. This was discussed with Sally and incorporated in the "Master Plan". Emily was still being bullied at school and we looked at the "Invisible Armour" technique by way of a coping strategy.

Telephone contact
Emily postponed her next session because of a holiday. She was pleased to say that she was maintaining her progress, was feeling much better and that her weight continued steadily to increase.

Session 4
Five weeks later, Emily reported being able to eat a little more in the evenings. Family meals definitely helped. Her brother in particular was good at distracting her, which made her more relaxed and able to eat. She had been on holiday with her family and friends, which she had thoroughly enjoyed: "Much better than last year ... I could do what I wanted, I have so much more energy." She was enjoying her food more, having finally "woken up her taste buds", and was pleased about that. She had been able to have a McDonald's meal with her friends and felt much more included and "less of a freak now I've got some meat on me!" Her weight was now up by 5.5 kilos since starting treatment. She was able to do her paper round without getting out of puff. Most importantly, the bullying had stopped. She had found the "invisible armour" a scream. The bullies were so surprised when she did not react to their comments that they soon stopped having a go at her.

On the scale of 0-10 she felt "pretty much at Miracle Day level", at 8-9. Emily was eating regular meals and snacks and had increased her dinner portions by a small amount. Her schoolwork had improved and her teachers were pleased with her progress. The school holidays had started and she was having a good time with her friends. At home, her parents had been "getting on at her" less and even her brother was being nice. The cats were worn out because she played with them so much. Emily had progressed to the "action stage", reporting sustained progress and inventing new coping strategies between sessions. We arranged to meet again five weeks later, but her weigh-ins continued fortnightly.

Session 5
Emily looked fit and healthy. She had her hair dyed and cut (a present for her fourteenth Birthday) and her figure looked more rounded. She had put on another two kilos, bringing the total weight gain up to 7.5 kg, and now weighed 43.5 kg. Her

periods had re-commenced. Emily had mixed feelings about this, "because of the hassle", but said it pleased her mother as it showed her she was getting better. We reiterated her successes, celebrated her progress and looked at how far she had come. She continued to be at 8-9 on the scale, in spite of not enjoying school as much because of exam time. The bullying had completely stopped. As she was doing so well we cut the session short and agreed to meet again in six weeks.

Evaluation, session 5
Emily continued to improve and gain weight. Her increased food intake had given her energy and she had built her self-confidence to such a degree that the bullying, which had been a major contributory factor to her illness, had completely stopped. We did a little solution-focused work to help her stand up to the bullies (imagine you wear the invisible armour, what do you see yourself doing? What else? What will their reaction be? etc.) and this illustrates that it is not necessary to explore all the ins and outs of that negative experience. Instead we looked at what Emily would do and how she would feel when she coped better, which smoothed the way for her actually carrying out her plan of action.

Session 6
Emily's BMI had gone up to 19. She was still feeling well, and enthusiastic about some new projects at school. On average she felt 8-9 on the scale, but there were times she was at a solid 9.
Asked what she was getting up to these days, she said:
"Oh, loads of things.... I'm so busy! I have loads of energy, I'm eating well. I go out with my friends, shopping in town, or to the cinema. I play football and basketball. I have a lot of fun. I'm more happy and cheerful and my mum is happy now. Especially because I eat all sorts of new things now, and my periods are back. [Pulls face: laughter] I can eat anything I like now. And I look forward to going to school for the first time."

We considered what she could do if she felt herself slipping a bit. She thought she could put her invisible armour back on, and recognised that the first thing she would need to do was eat a bit more, because that immediately made her feel better. She would enlist the support of her friends, teachers and parents and we discussed that, if she needed to, she could ring the surgery for a top-up session with me.
I asked what advice she would give if she met someone in the same situation she had been in.
E: I'd say, if it was a bully trying to get you to feel small, stand up for yourself. You can do it. Increase your self-esteem!
T: What would you tell them to do that would increase their self-esteem?

E: I'd say, "Look at what you want to be like! Just feel sorry for those bullies, they need to get a life!" And I'd say, "Just try to eat a little more, that will make your body and your mind stronger, and you will be able to stand up to them more."

We compared the notes I made from Emily's Miracle Day with the way she was feeling now, and she said she "regularly jumps for joy'". She had achieved everything she had imagined herself doing on the Miracle Day, and said it had made her even happier than she could have imagined. Evaluating the work we had done together, she rated therapy at 10. She had found the scales very useful, and coming to talk to someone who "really understood her" had been great. She had also liked the session with her mum, because it helped their relationship: Sally had been much more relaxed and subsequently Emily had started trying some new foods her mum had cooked for the family.

We agreed to finish therapy, but for the time being her weight would be monitored monthly and I would see her again in three months to catch up.

Follow-up session
Emily now felt at a steady 9. She felt strong and healthy, able to do anything she wanted, and the bullying had not returned. Her BMI was 19.5. I arranged for her to be weighed bimonthly and offered to see her in the future, should she ever need it.

Six months later
I telephoned to ask Emily's permission to write this case study. She readily agreed, and reported sustained recovery. The GP, Emily, Sally and I agreed that the bimonthly weigh-ins could now stop, but we would all stay vigilant in case the eating disorder decided to sneak up again.

5.

ANY QUESTIONS?

The following section is a collection of questions I am most commonly asked, and the answers are based on what I have learned from my clients and those who support them.

Is it true that people with eating disorders don't fully recover?
I think we need to establish the difference between "full recovery" and "getting better". My records show that most clients make significant changes during therapy, and continue to improve even after therapy has finished. If they start at 2 on the scale of 0-10, and end up at 8, this must mean that they have managed to "get better" or to "improve".

Now, to me, making a "full recovery" is a different kettle of fish, and a complicated one. The starting point on which to base "full recovery" must be to establish, "What is normal?" In terms of food, can we give a rule that serves everyone? What is normal for one person could be three square meals a day, whereas someone else might function better on six evenly spaced, smaller portions. Some people may eat more at weekends and less during the week, while others would never indulge in the occasional "blowout".

Because everyone needs food to eat, at times it is normal to think about what, where and when to have something to eat (or not). When people are well into recovery, this process will no longer cause anxiety, but they may still carry with them an awareness of what they have been through. They may recognise stresses and strains that would previously have made them behave in an eating-disordered way. Would that be abnormal? Would that mean they have not, and indeed never will fully recover? I cannot give you a concrete answer to this question, but I hope this book has proved that people do have the ability to "get better".

Are there particular clients you cannot work with?
My philosophy is this: where there is life there is hope. However dire the circumstances, there is always room for improvement. The client and I decide if the work I can offer will be of benefit. I make an agreement that if the condition gives me cause

for concern, I reserve the right to stop our work at least until it has improved. For instance, if the BMI drops to a dangerously low level, I will stop seeing a client until weight is re-gained, because at that point the brain is not well enough to engage in the work we do. Carrying on would waste money and time, which I think would be unethical.

When clients are seriously ill it is unsafe to work with them in isolation, so the help from other health professionals must be sought. Working alongside a like-minded nutritionist, as I have the good fortune to be able to do at times, promotes safe practice and can speed up the recovery rate.

How do you cope with such a resistant client group?
I don't like having that "R" word in my vocabulary at all. If a client appears to be "resistant", it is a sure-fire sign that I have not engaged with the client: I may have asked the wrong question or tried to use an unsuitable intervention, I've gone too fast, or I have not understood where they are coming from. The client usually responds with a "Yeah, but ..." so I apologise for getting it wrong, and ask them to put me back on track.

Do you suffer from burnout?
No. I think you are less likely to burn out if you focus on clients' strengths and coping strategies. Giving compliments and celebrating successes are energising activities, which can be engaged in however despondent a client may be. As with all therapies it is of course important to look after yourself: the client's eating disorder may be out to get you, too, so don't forget to put on the invisible armour. I think it is important to set firm boundaries around one's responsibilities as a therapist, and ensure safe and ethical practice by enlisting the help of other professionals, if need be seeking regular supervision, keeping the case load manageable, pursuing plenty of outside interests and taking regular holidays.

What do you do when a client has other problems too, e.g. self-harm or cutting?
I work on the premise that recovery is highly infectious. Therefore, if we work on one area, other problems will improve too. To make the work more focused I invite clients to choose what difficulty they want to address. So if we deal with the eating disorder, the cutting is treated "by proxy".

I take a position of "not knowing": "Tell me what is useful about it.... How does your eating disorder help you? What does it enable you to do differently?" In general, the usefulness of the behaviour is immediate stress relief, but most clients eventually conclude that the long-term benefits are illusory. As a client recognises the meagre benefits of an eating problem, and starts to look for alternative ways of handling stress, the cutting too will become less necessary.

How long does it take for people to recover?
How long is a piece of string? It depends on the type of eating disorder, how badly affected a client is, how motivated he or she is to overcome it, and an individual's perception of what recovery looks like. Some clients have an eating disorder most of their lives and manage to tick along reasonably well in spite of it. Others have a much lower "monster-tolerance level" and are able to rid themselves of the problem very quickly.

How many sessions do your clients normally have?
Another piece of string! The required amount of sessions varies, and depends on a multitude of facets: the severity of the eating distress, the support structure outside therapy and the stage of recovery at which a client commenced therapy, to name but a few. Some clients need only one or two sessions, while those recovering from chronic disorders need much more. However many sessions a client decides to have, I check the usefulness of our work at the end of every session and extend and invitation to make another appointment. The client decides how far apart these sessions need to be. Frequently, clients see me for three or four weekly sessions and then begin to lengthen the intervals to weekly, three-weekly and then monthly intervals.

Is solution-focused therapy just a "plaster on the wound"?
Read my book!

(Teacher:) I think a pupil in my class has an eating disorder. What should I do?
A lot of people wonder about this, so I make a point of asking my younger clients how teachers have been helpful in their recovery. Many of them agree that a useful approach was for the teacher to come alongside the person, gently voicing concerns – something like, "I hope you don't mind us having this chat, and I may be totally wrong, but you seem to have lost/gained a lot of weight recently. I just wanted you to know that if there is a problem, if you'd like to talk to me in confidence, then this can be arranged." It might help to have some information from the Eating Disorders Association to give out. People may always flatly deny that there is a problem (a sign of the pre-contemplative phase described earlier) but at least you will have sown a seed and made the first contact.

Many schools address eating disorders as part of their curriculum, and when I talk to groups I always start by saying, "The subject we are going to look at may touch a nerve with someone, because you know about eating disorders from your own experience, or you know someone who is suffering. If this is the case, please feel free to ask questions during the session, or come and talk to me or your teacher in confidence afterwards." This gives pupils the opportunity to talk, but it is their responsibility to decide if the moment feels right.

If you continue to be concerned about a pupil, but he or she does not respond to your overtures, don't be disheartened. Many people tell me they did appreciate the interest and the support that was offered, but at that time they were so entrenched that they were not able to respond. Eventually the penny may drop, but only when the person is ready.

(Youth worker:) I work with teenagers and one of them told me she throws up regularly. Should I tell her parents?
Before taking action I would talk it through with her, because she may not want her parents to know about it (at least not yet). You could give her a choice: "What would you like me to do with this information: keep it confidential or have a chat with your parents?" or, "What do you think you could do to improve things?" These are questions that immediately spring to mind. Set safe boundaries for yourself, telling her that if you are seriously concerned about her welfare, you may have to break the confidence.

(Parent:) Is it my fault that my child has an eating disorder?
There is never a single cause in an eating disorder. The relationship between parent and child may be a contributory factor in some cases, but I find that people with eating disorders can equally come from stable, loving homes, and have siblings who do not suffer. There are many different aspects that will, when combined, cause an eating disorder to erupt.

Your child's eating disorder can thrive on your feelings of guilt, making you focus on the times when you fall out, when you've let her down, when you could have done better. You could go down that slippery slope but, alternatively, you could look at the times you support her, love her, care for her, and let her know that you are there to help her get through this difficult, confusing time.

(Person contemplating recovery:) I have been told that I have anorexia, but I don't believe the doctor because I weigh too much.
The media equate anorexia nervosa with skeletal imagery. People of such low body weight are likely to have suffered for a very long time, and are virtually dead on their feet. Thinking that an eating disorder can be diagnosed by weight is dangerous because many people are very seriously ill even at a reasonable weight. Because they look "normal", they are not considered in need of help. Consequently, immense suffering goes on unnecessarily.

Many equally important factors must be considered. We would need to check if you have regular menstrual periods, how you feel about yourself, what your confidence is like, what your interests are, whether you are happy with your energy level, what you generally think about, if you are satisfied with your weight and body-shape, whether you enjoy a full social life, and whether you able to cope with work/school, are you generally even-tempered, etc. Your views give a broad picture of what is going on, and on that basis appropriate support can be offered to start making some improvements.

(Husband:) My wife has bulimia, she says I don't care and I don't understand her. How can I help her?
This is a classic accusation. The answer to that is, you obviously *do* care, otherwise why would you be here asking me this question?

Start looking for exceptions. When does she see that you do care? When was the last time you successfully showed her you cared? What did you do? Can you do more of it? What will she notice? What will her reaction be?

In terms of "not understanding her", if you do not have personal experience, or have not worked closely with those in eating distress, it is very difficult to understand what is a very complex problem. But with her help you can get closer than you are now. What could you do show her that you are willing to increase your understanding? What difference will this make? What are you already doing in order to understand her better? (For example, coming to this information evening, reading books and leaflets, watching programmes on TV about the topic.) It may be useful for you to know that many of my clients say they felt most understood when they were able to talk to a good listener; that is, someone who did not immediately give advice or try to sort out their problem for them. Would it be worth checking this with your wife?

(Parents:) Our daughter has an eating disorder and we just can't do anything right at the moment. The slightest thing and she bites our heads off. What can we do?
It is the monster that has managed to persuade you that you can't do *anything* right. It must have knocked your self-confidence something rotten. In solution-focused terms we could ask questions such as, "What are the times that things are a little better? What is it like when you *do* get a little something right?"

It is very frightening to see the enormous changes that occur when eating disorders get a hold. Chaotic eating causes a chaotic mindset, so in practical terms it would be good if your daughter could be persuaded to eat small, regular meals. Ask her what she will be able to eat and slowly try to build on that.

If your child could agree with you that a monster has attached itself to her and is making her behave unreasonably, you can start forming an alliance with her against it, rather than, as your child perceives the situation, you working against her. So when she flies off the handle you can say (or think), "This is not my lovely daughter, it's her monster. What can we do to get it off her shoulder?" Also, monitor very carefully what is going on when her behaviour is a little better. What is different? What is she doing? What are you doing? Can you do some more of what has made the difference?

(Mother:) My son is so unpredictable. He eats low fat strawberry yoghurts from "X" supermarket all the time, but when I came home with some more he exploded because they were the wrong flavour!
Eating disorders make people fickle and unpredictable. I know it's hard, but try not to be crushed by this. You are doing your best, trying to please him by getting exactly the right food, and the next thing you know, you're virtually wearing that yoghurt. His mood swings probably have nothing to do with the flavour of the yoghurt at all; rather, the monster is spoiling for a fight, in order to push another wedge between you.

It is not necessary to accept rude behaviour, so (try to) stay calm and state the facts: you were only doing your best, you had not realised he had gone off these yoghurts, you'd appreciate fair warning before you invest in six yoghurts next time, and what would he like instead? Alternatively, invite him to buy his own.

(Parents:) Our teenager is terribly rude, but we dare not discipline her because that might make her eating disorder worse.
Is she rude because of her age, or because of her eating disorder? When was she less rude? When was the last time you were able to curb her rudeness? What did you do? Can you do more of it? Monsters love to cause havoc in families. My clients have said that it is helpful to set down firm rules as to what is, and what is not, acceptable. If you tread on eggshells around her it means the eating disorder has won, which will definitely make matters worse.

(Someone who has recovered:) I suffered from an eating disorder but now that I am better I would like to work as a volunteer to help other people overcome their problems. How do I go about this?
I am often asked this question, not only by people who have overcome an eating disorder, but also by those who have cared for someone with such a problem. Helping others with a complaint of which you have first-hand knowledge can be a healing experience.

The Eating Disorders Association (see reference at the back of this book) will be able to give you information. They run a network of self-help groups all over the country and provide training and support for group leaders. They state that those wishing to get involved in a leading capacity must have been recovered for at least eighteen months. This is to prevent being drawn back into the eating disorder by others who suffer in a similar way. I would add to this that if you consider helping people in eating distress in a structured way (a self-help group, chat line, therapy, counselling etc.) it is essential to have supervision, particularly if you have had the illness yourself, or if you have supported a close relative or friend.

(Friend:) I think my friend has a problem with food. She eats in secret, but I know because I find wrappers tucked out of sight, and she's put on loads of weight. Do I challenge her or is it better to stay silent? I'm so afraid I may offend her.
Let her know that you think she may have a problem. Invite her to talk about it to you. If she flatly denies that anything is wrong, let her know that you are there to support her if she needs it. If she does want to talk, devise a plan between you that will help her take her mind off food. You could get some information about binge eating to help increase your understanding, or you could gently suggest she gets some professional help.

(Wife:) My husband eats all the time. He has been called clinically obese. What do you suggest I do?
What do you already do that makes a little difference? Can you do more of that? And, most importantly, does he actually want to stop eating? If he does not see any benefit in reducing his weight, you will not be able to persuade him. Are you the only person trying to help him, or is there anyone else he could turn to for support?

Your question does conjure up a strange picture. It makes me want to find out things such as, does he really eat all the time? How does he stop eating (e.g. when he goes to bed)? How does he decide to go stop eating and go to bed? Are there times he eats less? Are there times that he chooses not to eat something? Is there anything he'd rather be doing than eating?

My clients often say that they feel totally out of control, so we look for exceptions. That is, the times they show (even tiny) signs of control. For instance, when they ate only four chocolate bars instead of six, or when they decided to leave half the tub of ice cream for later, or when they wanted to eat but decided to do something else first. This shows clients that they do make decisions, and we then try and do more of what works. It may be an idea to have some blood tests done to exclude hormone imbalance. Some of my clients have benefited from dietary advice and/or medication.

(Parents:) It is so difficult living with an eating disorder. We used to go out for meals regularly, but now our son is an anorexic we can't do that anymore.
It sounds like the monster is ruling the roost. It's got so big that it's taken over your child completely. Parents have told me that things get easier when they try and live life as normally as possible. In other words, if you used to go out regularly with your family and enjoyed it, then carry on doing it. Even if it is less enjoyable then before, try and make it as good as you can, or if that is not possible, just pretend that you're enjoying it. You could try to give your child fair warning of what is going to happen, and invite him to come with you. He might need reassurance that if he does decide to join you, you will not make a fuss of what he does or does not eat, and that having the pleasure of his company would be greatly appreciated. Alternatively, he is welcome to stay at home and you won't argue over that.

(Friend:) I can see that my friend has a problem, but every time I try to talk to her about it, she shuts me out.
Eating disorders thrive on secrecy. As long as they can convince the sufferer that there is nothing wrong, they can stave off the threat of a helping hand. After all, where would the monster be if the sufferer decided to get better? You are a real threat to the eating disorder and if your friend manages to continue shutting you out, you may finally give up and leave her to it, which will create more time and space for the eating disorder to develop. So it is good that you have voiced your concerns, that you can let her eating disorder know that it's been rumbled. Bit by bit, she may get to recognise it too, but it may take a long time, and it may test your patience.

I guess that in the end it is your friend's privilege to decide what is and what is not problematic for her. It is also her responsibility to look after her own health. Keep supporting her if you can, as many clients tell me that although they may not have shown much appreciation at the time, having faithful friends alongside them in their "pre-contemplative" phase was a tremendous comfort.

And finally …
I hope that I have conveyed some aspects of the solution-focused philosophical stance towards clients: its sense of equality, a curiosity to find out how things work for them, respectfully inviting them to consider change, giving hope and encouragement, and approaching their treatment by way of "leading from behind", which many clients have said was particularly helpful.

Alongside this there is the value of practical interventions, such as looking for exceptions, client-led goal setting, taking small achievable steps to move further along the scale, and complimenting, to name but a few. It is this that attracted me to solution-focused therapy in the first place, and it is what most of my clients respond to by making the longed-for changes to improve their lives.

There are many more things I would like to have said, many stories I would like to have told, but sadly there are no more pages left. However, I hope this book has gone some way to explode the myth that people with eating disorders are "impossible to work with". I am off to do more of what works, and wish you every success as you do the same!

BIBLIOGRAPHY

Abraham, S. and Llewellyn-Jones, D. (1984), *Eating Disorders, The Facts*. Oxford: Oxford University Press.
American Psychiatric Association (1987, 3rd Edition, Revised), *Diagnostic and Statistical manual of Mental Disorders*. Washington DC: American Psychiatric Association.
Beales, D. and Dolton, R.(2000). Eating disordered patients: personality, alexithymia and implications for primary care. *British Journal of General Practice*, vol.50, pp. 21-26.
Berg, I. K. (1993), *Family preservation, A Brief Therapy Workbook*. London: Brief Therapy Press.
Bond, T. (1997), *Standards and Ethics for Counselling in Action*. London: Sage.
Bovey, S. (1984), *The Forbidden Body*. London: Penguin.
British Association of Counselling (1996), *Code of ethics and Practice for Counsellors*. Rugby: BAC Publications.
Bruch, H. (1974), *Eating Disorders – Obesity, Anorexia Nervosa and the Person Within*. London: Routledge & Kegan-Paul.
Bruch, H. (1978), *The Golden Cage: The Enigma of Anorexia Nervosa*. London: Open Books.
Carlat, D. J. and Camargo, C. A. (1991), Review of Bulimia Nervosa in Males. *American Journal of Psychiatry*, Vol. 148, part 7, pp. 831-842.
Dolan, Y. (1991), *Resolving Sexual Abuse* New York: Norton.
Eating Disorders Association (EDA), (2000), *Document: Eating Disorders, The need for action in 2000 and beyond*. Norwich: Eating Disorders Association.
European Eating Disorders Review, Volume 8, Number 3, March 2000. Chichester: J. Wiley & Sons.
Fairburn, C. (1995), *Overcoming Binge Eating*. London: Guilford Press.
Foucault, M. (1973), *The Birth of a Clinic: an Archaeology of Medical Perception*. London: Tavistock.
Friedman, S. (ed) (1993) *The New language of Change: Constructive Collaboration in Psychotherapy*. New York: Guildford Press.
George, E.; Iveson, C., and Ratner, H. (1999), *Problem to Solution*. London: Brief Therapy Press.
Grayling, A.C. (1996), *Wittgenstein*. Oxford: Open University Press.
Grogan, S. (1999), *Body Image*. London: Routledge.
Hepworth, J. (1999), *The Social Construction of Anorexia Nervosa*. London: Sage.
McFarland, B. (1995) *Brief Therapy and Eating Disorders: a Practical Guide to Solution-Focused Work with Clients*. San Francisco: Jossey-Bass.
Miller, S., Hubble, M. and Duncan, B. (1996), *Handbook of Solution-Focused Brief Therapy*. San

Francisco: Jossey-Bass.

Miller, S.; Hubble, M. and Duncan, B. (1995), *Escape from Babel*. New York: W.W.Norton.

Miller, S., Hubble,M. and Duncan, B. (1997), *Psychotherapy with "Impossible Cases"*. New York: W.W. Norton.

National Mental Health Framework Document (1999), Modern Standards and Services Model.

O'Connell, B. (1998), *Solution-Focused Therapy*. London: Sage.

O'Hanlon, W. and Beadle, S. (1997), *A Field Guide to Possibility Land: Possibility Therapy methods*. London: Brief Therapy Press.

O'Hanlon, W. and Hudson, P. (1989), *Re-writing Love Stories: Brief Marital Therapy*. London: W.W. Norton.

Orbach, S. (1988), *Fat is a Feminist Issue*. London: Arrow.

Palmer, R. L. (1980), *Anorexia Nervosa – a guide for suffers and their families*. London: Penguin.

Palmer,R. and Treasure,J. (1999), Providing Specialist Services for Anorexia nervosa. *British Journal of Psychiatry*, vol. 175, pp. 306-309.

Prochasca, J. and DiClemente, C. (1984), *The Trans-theoretical Approach*. Homewood: Dow Jones Irwin.

Rabinow, P. (1986), *The Foucault Reader*. London: Penguin.

Robinson, P. (1998), A Holistic Approach to Eating Disorders. *Psychiatry in Practice*, Spring 1998, pp. 6-8.

deShazer, S. (1988), *Clues: Investigating Solutions in Brief Therapy*. San Francisco: Jossey-Bass.

Talmon, M. (1990), *Single Session Therapy*. San Francisco: Josey-Bass.

Treasure, J. (1997), *Anorexia Nervosa: a survival guide for families, friends and Sufferers*. Hove: Psychology Press.

Treasure, J. and Schmidt, U. (1998), Beyond Effectiveness and Efficiency Lies Quality in Service for Eating Disorders. *European Eating Disorders Review*, Vol. 6, pp 1-17.

Treasure, J., Ward, A. (1997), A Practical Guide to the Use of Motivational Interviewing, *European Eating Disorders Review*, Vol. 5, pp. 102-114.

Treasure, J. (1999), Anorexia Nervosa and Bulimia Nervosa, *Prescriber's Journal* Vol.39, no. 4, pp. 227-233.

Warde, A. (1997), *Consumption, Food & Taste*. London: Sage.

White, C. and Denborough, D. (1990), *Introducing Narrative Therapy* Adelaide: Dulwich Press.

White, M. and Epson, D. (1990), *Narrative Means to Therapeutic Ends*. London: Norton.

White, M. (1997), *Narratives of Therapists' Lives*. Adelaide: Dulwich Press.

White, M. (1998), *Re-Authoring Lives*. Adelaide: Dulwich Publications.

Useful addresses:

Information about eating disorders:
Eating Disorders Association
First Floor, Wensum House
103 Prince of Wales Road
Norwich
Norfolk NR1 1DW.
Admin: 01603 619090
Media: 01603 624310
Helpline: 01603 621414
Youth helpline: 01603 765050
Email: info@edauk.com
Website: www.edauk.com

Information about solution-focused brief therapy:
Brief Therapy Practice
4d Shirland Mews
London W9 3DY
Telephone: 020 8968 0070
Email: solutions@brieftherapy.org.uk
Website: www.brieftherapy.org.uk

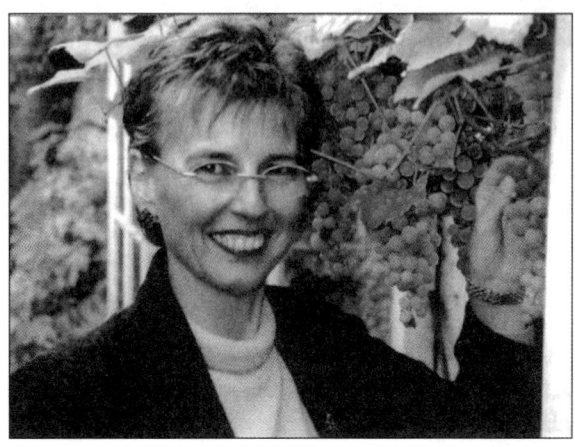

About the Author

Born in the 1950s in Holland, Frederike Jacob moved to England in 1977, where she met and married Nick in 1979. They have a teenage son and a daughter.

Frederike's background is in nursing and interior decorating, which came to an abrupt end in 1994 following a back injury. She felt she still had another career in her, decided to train as a counsellor, and specialised in eating disorders because she had noticed there was a distinct lack of professional help for those trying to recover. Originally trained psychodynamically, she was introduced to solution-focused therapy in 1997 and immediately began to incorporate the model into her practice. She discovered that not only did clients respond better to solution-focused therapy and made progress in a shorter time, but she also felt empowered by the process.

Frederike completed her MA Degree in Counselling Studies in August 2000 with a research project entitled, "Does Solution-Focused Therapy Help in the Recovery from Eating Disorders?" This showed that solution-focused therapy can have a significant role in overcoming the distress that is caused by the various forms of eating disorders.

She works in Ipswich, Suffolk, as a solution-focused therapist in private practice, general practice, and as co-facilitator of an eating disorder recovery group for the Local Health Trust. She gives talks and lectures and holds workshops at national and international level.

In her spare time she enjoys the company of her family and friends, painting, growing plants from seeds, arranging flowers, looking after the ancient vine in her greenhouse, travelling, giving and going to parties, hugging her cats, bicycling and going for walks. Oh … and shopping!

One day the birds will sing...

by Melanie Wright

The day begins as any other –
I awake from my slumber snuggled deep in my duvet
as if a butterfly cocooned in my outer layer before I break free
and enter the world anew.

The world around me is warm and welcoming as I step out of bed and prepare for
    the first day of the rest of my life.
I shower - and realise my body shape does not worry me for the first time in ages.
I dress - and discover that I like the person smiling back at me from the mirror,
and I tuck into a breakfast of pancakes and maple syrup.

Suddenly it hits me - getting dressed is instinctive and quick,
rather than a constant search for reassurance and correcting of clothes.
My mirror appeared to have been swapped in the night,
From the fairground distorter it has been for so many years
to a simple reflector of the truth.

Later on, the task of driving to the shops takes less time
for the comfort needed from the mirrors within is absent.
And when there, I fly past the mirrored windows
with a strange lack of need to check myself
and hardly a glance at the glass alongside.

Before I know it is it time for dinner, and amazingly it hasn't been
pressing itself onto my mind ever since I last tasted food.
Even more odd is the feeling that I can have whatever I desire
without it being a problem.
The needless phone call becomes an exchange of loving statements,
rather than the desperate reassurance of days gone by.

But more importantly, my mind can focus on the job in hand.
Previously nothing but food would have filtered through,
but the channel seems to have widened,
and these thoughts caught in a sieve until
the appropriate time of day.

Suddenly now, things seem to attract my attention
which before would have drifted around the surface until forgotten.
Connections remade with friends of old,
and life turns back to a series of going out and staying in,
rather than staying in and staying in.
For my friend my fear has shrunk considerable from view.